Contributors

Audrey Knippa, MS, MPH, RN, CNE
Nursing Education Coordinator and
  Content Project Leader

Sheryl Sommer, PhD, MSN, RN
Director, Nursing Curriculum and
  Education Services

Brenda Ball, MEd, BSN, RN
Nursing Education Specialist

Lois Churchill, MN, RN
Nursing Education Specialist

Carrie B. Elkins, DHSc, MSN, PHCNS, BC
Nursing Education Specialist

Mary Jane Janowski, MA, BSN, RN
Nursing Resource Specialist

Karin Roberts, PhD, MSN, RN, CNE
Nursing Education Coordinator

Mendy G. Wright, DNP, MSN, RN
Nursing Education Specialist

Derek Prater, MS Journalism
Lead Product Developer and Editorial Project Leader

Erika A. Archer, BS Education, Foreign Language
Product Developer

Johanna Barnes, BA Journalism
Product Developer

Chris Crawford, BS Journalism
Product Developer

Hilary E. Groninger, BS Journalism
Product Developer

Megan E. Herre, BS Journalism
Product Developer

Amanda Lehman, BA English
Product Developer

Joanna Shindler, BA Journalism
Product Developer

Brant L. Stacy, BS Journalism, BA English
Product Developer

Consultants

Susan Adcock, MS, RN

Christina D. Brazier, MSN, RN

Phyllis M. Jacobs, MSN, RN

INTELLECTUAL PROPERTY NOTICE

IMPORTANT NOTICE TO THE READER

USER'S GUIDE

Welcome to the Assessment Technologies Institute® RN Mental Health Nursing Review Module Edition 8.0. The mission of ATI's Content Mastery Series® review modules is to provide user-friendly compendiums of nursing knowledge that will:

- Help you locate important information quickly.

- Assist in your remediation efforts.

- Provide exercises for applying your nursing knowledge.

- Facilitate your entry into the nursing profession as a newly licensed RN.

Organization

This review module is organized into units covering foundations for mental health nursing, traditional nonpharmacological therapies, psychobiologic disorders, psychopharmacological therapies, special populations, and psychiatric emergencies. Chapters within these units conform to one of four organizing principles for presenting the content:

- Nursing concepts

- Procedures

- Disorders

- Medications

Nursing concepts chapters begin with an overview describing the central concept and its relevance to nursing. Subordinate themes are covered in outline form to demonstrate relationships and present the information in a clear, succinct manner.

Procedures chapters include an overview describing the procedure(s) covered in the chapter. These chapters will provide you with nursing knowledge relevant to each procedure, including indications, interpretations of findings, client outcomes, nursing actions, and complications.

Disorders chapters include an overview describing the disorder. These chapters cover assessments, including risk factors, subjective data, and objective data, and collaborative care, including nursing care, medications, interdisciplinary care, therapeutic procedures, and client outcomes.

Medications chapters include an overview describing a disorder or group of disorders. Medications used to treat these disorders are grouped according to classification. A specific medication may be selected as a prototype or example of the characteristics of medications in this classification. These sections include information about how the medication works, its therapeutic uses, and routes of administration. Next, you will find information about complications, contraindications, and medication and food interactions, as well as nursing interventions and client education to help prevent and/or manage these issues. Finally, the chapter includes information on nursing administration of the medication and evaluation of the medication's effectiveness.

Application Exercises

Questions are provided at the end of each chapter so you can practice applying your knowledge. The Application Exercises include both NCLEX-style questions, such as multiple-choice and multiple-select items, and questions that ask you to apply your knowledge in other formats, such as short-answer and matching items. After the Application Exercises, an answer key is provided, along with rationales for the answers.

NCLEX® Connections

To prepare for the NCLEX-RN, it is important for you to understand how the content in this review module is connected to the NCLEX-RN test plan. You can find information on the detailed test plan at the National Council of State Boards of Nursing's Web site: https://www.ncsbn.org/. When reviewing content in this review module, regularly ask yourself, "How does this content fit into the test plan, and what types of questions related to this content should I expect?"

To help you in this process, we've included NCLEX Connections at the beginning of each unit and with each question in the Application Exercises Answer Keys. The NCLEX Connections at the beginning of each unit will point out areas of the detailed test plan that relate to the content within that unit. The NCLEX Connections attached to the Application Exercises Answer Keys will demonstrate how each exercise fits within the detailed content outline.

These NCLEX Connections will help you understand how the detailed content outline is organized, starting with major client needs categories and subcategories and followed by related content areas and tasks. The major client needs categories are:

- Safe and Effective Care Environment
    - Management of Care
    - Safety and Infection Control
- Health Promotion and Maintenance
- Psychosocial Integrity
- Physiological Integrity
    - Basic Care and Comfort
    - Pharmacological and Parenteral Therapies
    - Reduction of Risk Potential
    - Physiological Adaptation

An NCLEX Connection might, for example, alert you that content within a unit is related to:

- Psychosocial Integrity
    - Behavioral Interventions
        - Incorporate behavioral management techniques when caring for a client.

Icons

Icons are used throughout the review module to draw your attention to particular areas. Keep an eye out for these icons:

 This icon indicates an Overview, or introduction, to a particular subject matter. Descriptions and categories will typically be found in an Overview.

 This icon is used for the Application Exercises and the Application Exercises Answer Keys.

 This icon is used for NCLEX connections.

 This icon is used for gerontological content. When you see this icon, take note of information that is specific to aging or the care of older adult clients.

 This icon is used for content related to safety. When you see this icon, take note of safety concerns or steps that nurses can take to ensure client safety and a safe environment.

 This icon indicates that a media supplement, such as a graphic, an animation, or a video, is available. If you have an electronic copy of the review module, this icon will appear alongside clickable links to media supplements. If you have a hardcopy version of the review module, visit www.atitesting.com for details on how to access these features.

Feedback

ATI welcomes feedback regarding this review module. Please provide comments to: comments@atitesting.com.

Table of Contents

UNIT 1: FOUNDATIONS FOR MENTAL HEALTH NURSING

- Basic Mental Health Nursing Concepts
- Legal and Ethical Issues
- Effective Communication
- Anxiety and Defense Mechanisms
- Creating and Maintaining a Therapeutic and Safe Environment
- Diverse Practice Settings

NCLEX® CONNECTIONS

When reviewing the chapters in this unit, keep in mind the relevant sections of the NCLEX® outline, in particular:

CLIENT NEEDS: MANAGEMENT OF CARE

Relevant topics/tasks include:
- Advocacy
  - Utilize advocacy resources appropriately.
- Client Rights
  - Recognize the client's right to refuse treatment/procedures.
- Collaboration with Interdisciplinary Team
  - Collaborate with health care members in other disciplines when providing client care.
- Confidentiality/Information Security
  - Maintain the client's confidentiality/privacy.
- Ethical Practice
  - Recognize ethical dilemmas and take appropriate action.
- Legal Rights and Responsibilities
  - Identify legal issues affecting the client.

CLIENT NEEDS: SAFETY AND INFECTION CONTROL

Relevant topics/tasks include:
- Accident/Injury Prevention
  - Make an appropriate room assignment for the cognitively impaired client.
- Use of Restraints/Safety Devices
  - Monitor/evaluate the client's response to restraints/safety device.

UNIT 1	FOUNDATIONS FOR MENTAL HEALTH NURSING
Chapter 1	Basic Mental Health Nursing Concepts

Overview

- Provision of care to clients in mental health settings is based on standards of care set by the American Nurses Association, the American Psychiatric Nurses Association, and the International Society of Psychiatric-Mental Health Nurses. Foundational to this care is the use of the nursing process.

- Mental health nurses should use the nursing process, as well as a holistic approach (biological, social, psychological, and spiritual aspects) to care for clients in mental health settings.

- Various methods should be used to assess clients. These methods include observation, interviewing, physical examination, and collaboration.

Assessment

- Each encounter with a client involves an ongoing assessment.

- Psychosocial History

    o Perception of own health, beliefs about illness and wellness

    o Activity/leisure activities, how the client passes time

    o Use/abuse of substances

    o Stress level and coping abilities – usual coping strategies, support systems

    o Cultural beliefs and practices

    o Spiritual beliefs

- The Mental Status Examination (MSE)

View Media Supplement: Mental Status Examination (Video)

    o Level of consciousness may be described using the following terms, and observed behavior should be included in documentation:

        ▪ Alert

            □ The client is responsive and able to fully respond by opening her eyes and attending to a normal tone of voice and speech. She answers questions spontaneously and appropriately.

- Lethargy
  - The client is able to open her eyes and respond but is drowsy and falls asleep readily.
- Obtundation
  - The client needs to be lightly shaken to elicit a response, but she may be confused and slow to respond.
- Stupor
  - The client requires painful stimuli (pinching a tendon or rubbing the sternum) to elicit a brief response. She may not be able to respond verbally.
- Coma
  - No response can be achieved from repeated painful stimuli.
    - Abnormal posturing in the client who is comatose
    - Decorticate rigidity – flexion and internal rotation of upper-extremity joints and legs
    - Decerebrate rigidity – neck and elbow extension, wrist and finger flexion

○ Physical appearance

- Examination includes assessment of personal hygiene, grooming, and clothing choice. Expected findings with regard to this assessment are that the client is well-kept, clean, and dressed appropriately for the given environment.

○ Behavior

- Examination includes assessment of voluntary and involuntary body movements, and eye contact.
  - Mood
    - A client's mood provides information about the emotion that she is feeling.
  - Affect
    - A client's affect is an objective expression of mood, such as a flat affect or a lack of facial expression.

○ Cognitive and intellectual abilities

- Assess the client's orientation to time, person, and place.
- Assess the client's memory, both recent and remote.
  - Recent – Ask the client to repeat a series of numbers or a list of objects.
  - Remote – Ask the client to state a fact that is verifiable, such as his birth date or his mother's maiden name.
- Assess the client's level of knowledge. For example, ask him what he knows about his current illness or hospitalization.

- Assess the client's ability to calculate. For example, can he count backward from 100 in serials of 7?

- Assess the client's ability to think abstractly. For example, can he interpret a cliché, such as "A bird in the hand is worth two in the bush."? The ability to interpret this demonstrates a higher-level thought process.

- Perform an objective assessment of the client's perception of his illness.

- Assess the client's judgment based on his answer to a hypothetical question. For example, how would he answer the question, "What would you do if there were a fire in your room?" His response to the question should be logical.

- Assess the client's rate and volume of speech, as well as the quality of his language. His speech should be articulate and his responses meaningful and appropriate.

- Standardized Screening Tools

  o Mini-Mental State Examination

    - This examination is used to objectively assess a client's cognitive status by evaluating the following:

      □ Orientation to time and place

      □ Attention span and ability to calculate by counting backward by seven

      □ Registration and recalling of objects

      □ Language, including naming of objects, following of commands, and ability to write

  o Glasgow Coma Scale

    - This examination is used to obtain a baseline assessment of a client's level of consciousness, and for ongoing assessment. Eye, verbal, and motor response is evaluated, and a number value based on that response is assigned. The highest value possible is 15, which indicates that the client is awake and responding appropriately. A score of 3 indicates that the client is in a coma.

Considerations Across the Lifespan

- Children and Adolescents

  o Assessment includes temperament, social and environmental factors, cultural and religious concerns, and developmental level.

  o Mentally healthy children and adolescents should trust others, view the world as safe, accurately interpret their environments, master developmental tasks, and use appropriate coping skills.

  o Children and adolescents experience some of the same mental health problems as adults.

- Mental health and developmental disorders are not always easily diagnosed, and treatment interventions may be delayed or inadequate. Factors contributing to this include:
  - Lack of the ability or necessary skills to describe what is happening
  - A wide variation of "normal" behavior, especially in different developmental stages
- Assess this age group for mood, anxiety, developmental, behavioral, and eating disorders. Risk of suicide should also be considered.
- Use the standardized assessment tool, Home, Education/employment, peer group Activities, Drugs, Sexuality, and Suicide/depression (HEADSS) psychosocial assessment, to evaluate risk factors in the adolescent.

● **The Older Adult**

- In addition to the aforementioned assessments, a comprehensive assessment of the older adult client includes the following:
  - Functional ability, such as the ability to get up out of a chair
  - Economic and social status
  - Environmental factors, such as stairways in the home, that may affect the client's well-being and lifestyle
  - Physical assessment
- Standardized assessment tools that are specific to the older adult population, include:
  - Geriatric Depression Scale (short form)
  - Michigan Alcoholism Screening Test – Geriatric Version
  - Mini Mental Status Exam
  - Pain assessments including visual analogue scales, Wong-Baker FACES Pain Rating Scale, the McGill Pain Questionnaire (MPQ), and the Pain Assessment in Advanced Dementia (PAINAD) scale
- An assessment of all clients, including older adult clients, should be conducted in the following manner:
  - Use a private, quiet space with adequate lighting to accommodate for impaired vision and hearing.
  - Make an introduction, and determine the client's name preference
  - Stand or sit at the client's level to conduct the interview, rather than standing over a client who is bed bound or sitting in a chair.
  - Respect the client's personal space if he does not wish to be touched, but use touch to communicate caring as appropriate.
  - Be sure to include questions relating to difficulty sleeping, incontinence, falls or other injuries, depression, dizziness, and loss of energy.
  - Include the family and significant others as appropriate.

- Take a detailed medication history.

- Following the interview, summarize and ask for feedback from the client.

Mental Health Diagnoses

- The Diagnostic and Statistical Manual of Mental Disorders, 4th Edition, text revision (DSM-IV-TR), published by the American Psychiatric Association, is used as a diagnostic tool to identify medical diagnoses. It is used by mental health professionals for clients who have mental health disorders.

- Nurses use the DSM-IV-TR in the mental health setting to identify diagnoses and diagnostic criteria to guide assessment; identify nursing diagnoses; and to plan, implement, and evaluate care.

- Multiaxial System – The DSM-IV-TR uses a multiaxial system to assess clients in the mental health setting. It assesses for abnormal behavior, comorbid medical conditions, conditions within the environment, and level of functioning.

  o Axis I – all mental health diagnosis except for those found in Axis II

  o Axis II – any personality disorder diagnosis and mental retardation

  o Axis III – any general medical diagnosis, such as asthma

  o Axis IV – pertinent psychosocial problems and problems that may affect diagnosis, treatment, and prognosis of mental disorders

  o Axis V – global assessment of functioning (GAF) – an assessment of present and past-year functioning that rates the client's level of functioning in the areas of work performance, social abilities, and psychological ability on a scale of 1 to 100.

    - Scores of 80 to 100 generally indicate normal or near-normal function.

    - Scores of 60 to 80 indicate moderate problems.

    - Scores 40 and below indicate serious mental disability and/or functioning impairments.

    - Present and past-year GAF scores are compared to track the client's level of functioning. For example, a GAF of 50/80 indicates that the client presently has a GAF score of 50, with a previous score of 80 in the past year.

Therapeutic Strategies in the Mental Health Setting

MENTAL HEALTH NURSING INTERVENTIONS	
Counseling	• Using therapeutic communication skills • Assisting with problem solving • Crisis intervention • Stress management
Milieu therapy	• Orienting the client to the physical setting • Identifying rules and boundaries of the setting • Ensuring a safe environment for the client • Assisting the client to participate in appropriate activities
Promotion of self-care activities	• Offering assistance with self-care tasks • Allowing time for the client to complete self-care tasks • Setting incentives to promote client self-care
Psychobiological interventions	• Administering prescribed medications • Providing teaching to the client/family • Monitoring for side effects and effectiveness of therapy
Cognitive and behavioral therapies	• Modeling • Operant conditioning • Systematic desensitization
Health teaching	• Teaching social and coping skills
Health promotion and health maintenance	• Assisting the client with cessation of smoking • Monitoring other health conditions
Case management	• Coordinating holistic care to include medical, mental health, and social services

CHAPTER 1: BASIC MENTAL HEALTH NURSING CONCEPTS

(A) Application Exercises

1. While performing a mental status examination on a client, the nurse notices that the client's facial expression constantly appears angry. This information should be recorded as part of the client's

    A. behavior.

    B. appearance.

    C. affect.

    D. thought process.

2. During a mental status examination, a client who is hospitalized states that she is in the hospital "to help out with the other patients." The nurse should record this information as

    A. poor insight.

    B. decreased level of knowledge.

    C. decreased judgment.

    D. poor remote memory.

3. Which of the following are examples of subjective assessment data? (Select all that apply.)

    _____ "Client's speech is slow and soft."

    _____ "Client states he has no reason to live."

    _____ "Client is able to recall three numbers."

    _____ "Client meditates for relaxation."

    _____ "Client states that he drinks three beers a day."

4. A nurse is caring for a client diagnosed with paranoid schizophrenia, asthma, generalized anxiety disorder, and borderline personality disorder. Which of the following diagnoses should the nurse expect to find included in Axis II of this client's DSM-IV-TR axis diagnosis?

    A. Paranoid schizophrenia

    B. Asthma

    C. Generalized anxiety disorder

    D. Borderline personality disorder

5. A client is admitted to an acute care mental health facility. The following medical diagnoses and psychosocial information are available at the time of admission: hypothyroidism, mild mental retardation, bipolar I disorder. The client's highest level of functioning from a global assessment of functioning (GAF) performed a year ago was 45. Today, the highest level of functioning on the same scale is 15. The client has been fighting with other clients frequently at the group home. How should the nurse enter this information into the multiaxial system of the DSM- IV- TR?

Axis I:

Axis II:

Axis III:

Axis IV:

Axis V:

CHAPTER 1: BASIC MENTAL HEALTH NURSING CONCEPTS

 Application Exercises Answer Key

1. While performing a mental status examination on a client, the nurse notices that the client's facial expression constantly appears angry. This information should be recorded as part of the client's

    A. behavior.

    B. appearance.

    C. affect.

    D. thought process.

    Description of the client's facial expression is described as affect. Facial expression is not described in the areas of behavior, appearance, or thought process.

 NCLEX® Connection: Psychosocial Integrity, Mental Health Concepts

2. During a mental status examination, a client who is hospitalized states that she is in the hospital "to help out with the other patients." The nurse should record this information as

    A. poor insight.

    B. decreased level of knowledge.

    C. decreased judgment.

    D. poor remote memory.

    The nurse's objective assessment of the client's insight reflects the client's understanding of her current situation and medical condition. Knowledge, judgment, and memory are other objective cognitive assessments. None reflect the client's understanding of the responsibility for, or analysis of, the current situation.

 NCLEX® Connection: Psychosocial Integrity, Mental Health Concepts

3. Which of the following are examples of subjective assessment data? (Select all that apply.)

    _____ "Client's speech is slow and soft."

    __X__ **"Client states he has no reason to live."**

    _____ "Client is able to recall three numbers."

    __X__ **"Client meditates for relaxation."**

    __X__ **"Client states that he drinks three beers a day."**

    Subjective data includes psychosocial information about the client's thoughts, actions and feelings that can only be described by the client. Objective data is based on observable or verifiable facts.

 NCLEX® Connection: Psychosocial Integrity, Mental Health Concepts

4. A nurse is caring for a client diagnosed with paranoid schizophrenia, asthma, generalized anxiety disorder, and borderline personality disorder. Which of the following diagnoses should the nurse expect to find included in Axis II of this client's DSM-IV-TR axis diagnosis?

    A. Paranoid schizophrenia

    B. Asthma

    C. Generalized anxiety disorder

    D. Borderline personality disorder

    Personality disorders and mental retardation are included in Axis II. Paranoid schizophrenia and generalized anxiety disorder are found in Axis I. Asthma and other general medical conditions are found in Axis III.

    (N) **NCLEX® Connection: Psychosocial Integrity, Mental Health Concepts**

5. A client is admitted to an acute care mental health facility. The following medical diagnoses and psychosocial information are available at the time of admission: hypothyroidism, mild mental retardation, bipolar I disorder. The client's highest level of functioning from a global assessment of functioning (GAF) performed a year ago was 45. Today, the highest level of functioning on the same scale is 15. The client has been fighting with other clients frequently at the group home. How should the nurse enter this information into the multiaxial system of the DSM-IV-TR?

    Axis I: **Bipolar I disorder**

    Axis II: **Mild mental retardation**

    Axis III: **Hypothyroidism**

    Axis IV: **Has been fighting with other clients frequently at group home**

    Axis V: **GAF 15/45**

    Axis I includes most mental health clinical disorders, except those placed on Axis II. Axis II disorders include personality disorders and mental retardation. Axis III includes general medical disorders and problems. Axis IV includes pertinent psychosocial information or problems with living conditions. Axis V includes GAF for present assessment and previous assessment within 1 year of present.

    (N) **NCLEX® Connection: Psychosocial Integrity, Mental Health Concepts**

UNIT 1	FOUNDATIONS FOR MENTAL HEALTH NURSING
Chapter 2	Legal and Ethical Issues

(a) Overview

- A nurse who works in the mental health setting is responsible for practicing ethically, competently, safely, and in a manner consistent with all local, state, and federal laws.

- Nurses must have an understanding of ethical principles and how they apply when providing care for clients in mental health settings.

- Nurses are responsible for understanding and protecting client rights.

Legal Rights of Clients in the Mental Health Setting

- Clients who have been diagnosed and/or hospitalized with a mental health disorder are guaranteed the same civil rights as any other citizen. These include:

  o The right to humane treatment and care, such as medical and dental care

  o The right to vote

  o The right to due process of law, including the right to press legal charges against another person

- Clients also have various specific rights, including:

  o Informed consent and the right to refuse treatment

  o Confidentiality

  o A written plan of care/treatment that includes discharge follow-up, as well as participation in the care plan and review of that plan

  o Communication with persons outside the mental health facility, including family members, attorneys, and other health care professionals

  o Provision of adequate interpretive services if needed

  o Care provided with respect, dignity, and without discrimination

  o Freedom from harm related to physical or pharmacologic restraint, seclusion, and any physical or mental abuse or neglect

  o Provision of care with the least restrictive interventions necessary to meet the client's needs without allowing him to be a threat to himself or others

- Some legal issues regarding health care may be decided in court using a specialized civil category called a tort. A tort is a wrongful act or injury committed by an entity or person against another person or another person's property. Torts can be used to decide liability issues, as well as intentional issues that may involve criminal penalties, such as abuse of a client.

- State laws may vary greatly. The nurse must be aware of specific laws regarding client care within the state or states in which the nurse practices.

Ethical Issues for Clients in the Mental Health Setting

- In comparison to laws, statutes, and regulations (enacted by local, state, or federal government), ethical issues are philosophical ideas regarding right and wrong.

- Nurses are frequently confronted with ethical dilemmas regarding client care (bioethical issues).

- Since ethics are philosophical and involve values and morals, there is frequently no clear-cut simple resolution to an ethical dilemma.

- Ethical principles must be used to decide ethical issues. These include:

ETHICAL PRINCIPLE	DEFINITION	EXAMPLE
Beneficence	This relates to the quality of doing good and can be described as charity.	A nurse helps a newly admitted client with psychosis feel safe in the environment of the mental health facility.
Autonomy	This refers to the client's right to make his own decisions. But the client must accept the consequences of those decisions. The client must also respect the decisions of others.	Rather than giving advice to a client who has difficulty making decisions, a nurse helps the client explore all alternatives and arrive at a choice.
Justice	This is defined as fair and equal treatment for all.	During a treatment team meeting, a nurse leads a discussion regarding whether or not two clients who broke the same facility rule were treated equally.
Fidelity	This relates to loyalty and faithfulness to the client and to one's duty.	A client asks a nurse to be present when she talks to her mother for the first time in a year. The nurse remains with the client during this interaction.

ETHICAL PRINCIPLE	DEFINITION	EXAMPLE
Veracity	This refers to being honest when dealing with a client.	A client states, "You and that other staff member were talking about me, weren't you?" The nurse truthfully replies, "We were discussing ways to help you relate to the other clients in a more positive way."

Confidentiality

- The client's right to privacy is protected by the Health Insurance Portability and Accountability Act (HIPAA) of 2003.

- It is important to gain an understanding of the federal law and of various state laws as they relate to confidentiality in specific health care facilities.

- Information about the client, verbal and in writing, must only be shared with those who are responsible for implementing the client's treatment plan.

- Information may be shared with other persons not involved in the client treatment plan by client consent only.

- Specific mental health issues include disclosing HIV status, the duty to warn and protect third parties, and the reporting of child and elder abuse.

Resources for Solving Ethical Client Issues

- Code of Ethics for Nurses, found at http://nursingworld.org/

- Patient Care Partnership, found at http://www.aha.org/

- The nurse practice act of a specific state

- Legal advice from attorneys

- Facility policies

- Other members of the health care team, including facility bioethics committee (if available)

- Members of the clergy and other spiritual or ethical counselors

Types of Commitment to a Mental Health Facility

- Voluntary commitment – The client or client's guardian chooses commitment to a mental health facility in order to obtain treatment. A voluntarily committed client has the right to apply for release at any time. This client is considered competent, and so has the right to refuse medication and treatment.

- Involuntary (civil) commitment – The client enters the mental health facility against her will for an indefinite period of time. The commitment is based on the client's need for psychiatric treatment, the risk of harm to self or others, or the inability to provide self-care. The need for commitment could be determined by a judge of the court or by another agency. The number of physicians, which is usually two, required to certify that the client's condition requires commitment, varies from state to state.

  ○ Emergency involuntary commitment – a type of involuntary commitment in which the client is hospitalized to prevent harm to self or others. Emergency commitment is usually temporary (may be up to 10 days). This type of commitment is usually imposed by primary care providers, mental health providers, or police officers.

  ○ Observational or temporary involuntary commitment – a type of involuntary commitment in which the client is in need of observation, a diagnosis, and a treatment plan. The time for this type of commitment is controlled by state statute and varies greatly between states. This may be imposed by a family member, legal guardian, primary care provider, or a mental health provider.

  ○ Long-term or formal involuntary commitment – a type of commitment that is similar to temporary commitment but must be imposed by the courts. Time of commitment varies, but is usually 60 to180 days. Sometimes, there is no set release date.

  ○ Clients admitted under involuntary commitment are still considered competent and have the right to refuse treatment, unless they have gone through a legal competency hearing and have been judged incompetent. The client who has been judged incompetent has a temporary or permanent guardian, usually a family member if possible, appointed by the court. The guardian can sign informed consent for the client. The guardian is expected to consider what the client would want if he were still competent.

Ⓢ Client Rights Regarding Seclusion and Restraint

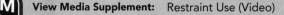

Ⓜ View Media Supplement: Restraint Use (Video)

- Nurses must know and follow federal/state/facility policies that govern the use of restraints.

- Use of seclusion rooms and/or restraints may be warranted and authorized for clients in some cases.

- In general, seclusion and/or restraint should be ordered for the shortest duration necessary, and only if less restrictive measures are not sufficient. They are for the physical protection of the client and/or the protection of other clients and staff.

- A client may voluntarily request temporary seclusion in cases where the environment is disturbing or seems too stimulating.

- Restraints can be either physical or chemical, such as neuroleptic medication to calm the client.

- Seclusion and/or restraint must never be used for:

    ○ Convenience of the staff

    ○ Punishment of the client

    ○ Clients who are extremely physically or mentally unstable

    ○ Clients who cannot tolerate the decreased stimulation of a seclusion room

- When all other less restrictive means have been tried to prevent a client from harming self or others, the following must occur in order for seclusion or restraint to be used:

    ○ The treatment must be ordered by the primary care provider in writing.

    ○ The order must specify the duration of treatment.

    ○ The provider must rewrite the order, specifying the type of restraint, every 24 hr or the frequency of time specified by facility policy.

    ○ Nursing responsibilities must be identified in the protocol, including how often the client should be:

        ▪ Assessed (including for safety and physical needs), and the client's behavior documented

        ▪ Offered food and fluid

        ▪ Toileted

        ▪ Monitored for vital signs

    ○ Complete documentation includes a description of the following:

        ▪ Precipitating events and behavior of the client prior to seclusion or restraint

        ▪ Alternative actions taken to avoid seclusion or restraint

        ▪ The time treatment began

        ▪ The client's current behavior, what foods or fluids were offered and taken, needs provided for, and vital signs

        ▪ Medication administration

- An emergency situation must be present for the charge nurse to use seclusion or restraints without first obtaining a provider's written order. If this treatment is initiated, the nurse must obtain the written order within a specified period of time (usually 15 to 30 min).

Tort Law in the Mental Health Setting

- Although intentional torts can occur in any health care setting, they are particularly likely to occur in mental health settings due to the increased likelihood of violence and client behavior that can be challenging to facility staff. Following are examples of torts:

INTENTIONAL TORT	EXAMPLE
False imprisonment	Confining a client to a specific area, such as a seclusion room, is false imprisonment if the reason for such confinement is for the convenience of the staff.
Assault	Making a threat to a client's person, such as approaching the client in a threatening manner with a syringe in hand, is considered assault.
Battery	Touching a client in a harmful or offensive way is considered battery. This would occur if the nurse threatening the client with a syringe actually grabbed the client and gave an injection.

Documentation

- It is vital to clearly and objectively document information related to violent or other unusual episodes. The nurse should document:
    - Client behavior in a clear and objective manner
        - Example: The client suddenly began to run down the hall with both hands in the air, screaming obscenities.
    - Staff response to disruptive, violent, or potentially harmful behavior, such as suicide threats or potential or actual harm to others, including timelines and the extent of response
        - Example: The client states, "I'm going to pound (other client) into the ground." Client has picked up a chair and is standing 3 ft from other client with chair held over his head in both hands. Nurse calls for help. Client is immediately told by nurse, "Put down the chair and back away from (the other person)." Other client moved away to safe area. Five other staff members respond to verbal call for help within 30 sec and stood several yards from client. Client then put the chair down, quietly turned around, walked to his room, and sat on the bed.

CHAPTER 2: LEGAL AND ETHICAL ISSUES

 Application Exercises

1. Which of the following is an example of a client who requires emergency admission to a mental health facility?

  A. A client with schizophrenia who has frequent hallucinations

  B. A client with symptoms of depression who attempted suicide a year ago

  C. A client with borderline personality disorder who assaulted a homeless man with a metal rod

  D. A client with bipolar disorder who paces quickly down the sidewalk while talking to himself

2. A client tells a student nurse, "Don't tell anyone, but I hid a sharp knife under my mattress in order to protect myself from my roommate, who is always yelling at me and threatening me." Which of the following actions should the nurse take?

  A. Keep the client's communication confidential, but talk to the client daily, using therapeutic communication to convince him to admit to hiding the knife.

  B. Keep the client's communication confidential, but watch the client and his roommate closely.

  C. Tell the client that this must be reported to health care staff, because it concerns the health and safety of the client and others.

  D. Report the incident, but do not inform the client of the intention to do so.

3. A nurse decides to put a client with psychosis in seclusion overnight because the unit is very short-staffed and the client frequently fights with other clients. This is an example of

  A. beneficence.

  B. a tort.

  C. a facility policy.

  D. justice.

4. A nurse is caring for a client in restraints. Which of the following is appropriate documentation? (Select all that apply.)

  _____ "Client ate most of his breakfast."

  _____ "Client was offered 8 oz of water every hr."

  _____ "Client shouted at assistive personnel."

  _____ "Client received chlorpromazine (Thorazine) 15 mg by mouth at 1000."

  _____ "Client acted out after lunch."

CHAPTER 2: LEGAL AND ETHICAL ISSUES

 Application Exercises Answer Key

1. Which of the following is an example of a client who requires emergency admission to a mental health facility?

   A. A client with schizophrenia who has frequent hallucinations

   B. A client with symptoms of depression who attempted suicide a year ago

   C. A client with borderline personality disorder who assaulted a homeless man with a metal rod

   D. A client with bipolar disorder who paces quickly down the sidewalk while talking to himself

   The client who is a current danger to self or others is a candidate for emergency admission. The presence of hallucinations, symptoms of depression without recent suicide attempt or intent to commit suicide, or other mental health symptoms does not constitute a clear reason for emergency commitment.

    NCLEX® Connection: Psychosocial Integrity, Crisis Intervention

2. A client tells a student nurse, "Don't tell anyone, but I hid a sharp knife under my mattress in order to protect myself from my roommate, who is always yelling at me and threatening me." Which of the following actions should the nurse take?

   A. Keep the client's communication confidential, but talk to the client daily, using therapeutic communication to convince him to admit to hiding the knife.

   B. Keep the client's communication confidential, but watch the client and his roommate closely.

   C. Tell the client that this must be reported to health care staff, because it concerns the health and safety of the client and others.

   D. Report the incident, but do not inform the client of the intention to do so.

   This is a serious safety issue that must be reported to staff. Using the principle of veracity, the student tells this client truthfully what must be done regarding the issue.

    NCLEX® Connection: Safety and Infection Control, Accident/Injury Prevention

3. A nurse decides to put a client with psychosis in seclusion overnight, because the unit is very short-staffed, and the client frequently fights with other clients. This is an example of

   A. beneficence.

   B. a tort.

   C. a facility policy.

   D. justice.

   A civil wrong that violates a client's civil rights is a tort, in this case, false imprisonment. The decision is neither beneficence (doing good for a client) nor justice (fair and equal treatment). If this were indeed a facility policy, it would certainly be violating a federal and state statute, and the nurse could still be held responsible for following it.

    NCLEX® Connection: Safety and Infection Control, Use of Restraints/Safety Devices

4. A nurse is caring for a client in restraints. Which of the following is appropriate documentation? (Select all that apply.)

	"Client ate most of his breakfast."
X	**"Client was offered 8 oz of water every hr."**
X	**"Client shouted at assistive personnel."**
X	**"Client received chlorpromazine (Thorazine) 15 mg by mouth at 1000."**
	"Client acted out after lunch."

Exactly how much water and how often it was offered, the description of the client's verbal communication, and the dosage and time of medication administration are all objective data that should be appropriately documented when a nurse is caring for a client in restraints. The facts that the client ate most of his breakfast and acted out over lunch are both subjective and should therefore not be documented.

(N) NCLEX® Connection: Safety and Infection Control, Use of Restraints/Safety Devices

UNIT 1	FOUNDATIONS FOR MENTAL HEALTH NURSING
Chapter 3	Effective Communication

Overview

- Communication is a complex process of sending, receiving, and comprehending messages between two or more people. It is a dynamic and ongoing process that creates a unique experience between the participants.

  o Communicating effectively is a skill that can be developed.

  o Nurses use communication when providing care to establish relationships, demonstrate caring, obtain information, and assist with changing behaviors.

  o Foundational to the nurse-client relationship is therapeutic communication.

Basic Communication

- Three Primary Levels of Basic Communication

  o Intrapersonal communication – communication that occurs within an individual. Also identified as "self-talk." This occurs within one's self and is the internal discussion that takes place when an individual is thinking thoughts and not outwardly verbalizing them. In nursing, intrapersonal communication allows the nurse to assess a client and/or situation and critically think about the client/situation before communicating verbally.

  o Interpersonal communication – communication that occurs between two or more people in a small group. This form of communication is the most common in nursing and requires an exchange of information with an individual or small group.

  o Public communication – communication that occurs within large groups of people. In nursing, this commonly occurs during educational endeavors where the nurse is teaching a large group of individuals, such as in a community setting.

  o Transpersonal communication – communication that addresses an individual's spiritual needs and provides interventions to meet those needs.

- Verbal Communication

VERBAL COMMUNICATION CONTENT OF THE MESSAGE	IMPACT ON THE COMMUNICATION
Vocabulary – These are the words that are used to communicate either a written or a spoken message.	Limited vocabulary or speaking a language other than English may make it difficult for the nurse to communicate with the client. Use of medical jargon may decrease client understanding.
Denotative/connotative meaning – When communicating, participants must share meanings.	Words that have multiple meanings may cause miscommunication if they are interpreted differently.
Clarity/brevity – The shortest, simplest communication is usually most effective.	Communication that is long and complex may be difficult to understand.
Timing/relevance – Knowing when to communicate allows the receiver to be more attentive to the message.	Communicating with a client who is in pain or distracted will make it difficult for the message to be conveyed.
Pacing – The rate of speech can communicate a meaning to the receiver.	Speaking rapidly may communicate the impression that the nurse is in a rush and does not have time for the client.
Intonation – The tone of voice can communicate a variety of feelings.	The nurse can communicate feelings, such as acceptance, judgment, and dislike through tone of voice.

- Nonverbal Communication

  - Nurses should be aware of how they communicate nonverbally. The nurse should assess the client's nonverbal communications for the meaning being conveyed, remembering that culture impacts interpretation. Attention to the following behaviors is important, as it is compared to the verbal message being conveyed:

    - Appearance

    - Posture

    - Gait

    - Facial expressions

    - Eye contact

    - Gestures

    - Sounds

    - Territoriality

    - Personal space

    - Silence

Therapeutic Communication

- Therapeutic communication is the purposeful use of communication to build and maintain helping relationships with clients, families, and significant others.

- The nurse uses interactive, purposeful communication skills to

  - elicit and attend to the client's thoughts, feelings, concerns, and needs.

  - express empathy and genuine concern for the client's and family's issues.

  - obtain information and give feedback about the client's condition.

  - intervene to promote functional behavior and effective interpersonal relationships.

  - evaluate the client's progress toward goals and outcomes.

- Children and older adults frequently require altered techniques to enhance communication.

- Use of the nursing process depends on therapeutic communication between the nurse, the client, the client's family, and the interdisciplinary care team.

- Characteristics of Therapeutic Communication

  - Client centered – not social or reciprocal

  - Purposeful, planned, and goal-directed

- Essential Components of Therapeutic Communication

  - Time – Plan for and allow adequate time to communicate.

  - Attending behaviors or active listening – These are nonverbal means of conveying interest in another.

    - Eye contact typically conveys interest and respect but varies by situation and culture.

    - Body language and posture may demonstrate level of comfort and ease.

    - Vocal quality enhances rapport and emphasizes particular topics or issues.

    - Verbal tracking provides feedback by restating or summarizing a client's statements.

  - Caring attitude – Show concern and facilitate an emotional connection with the client and the client's family.

  - Honesty – Be open, direct, truthful, and sincere.

  - Trust – Demonstrate reliability without doubt or question.

  - Empathy – Convey an objective awareness and understanding of the feelings, emotions, and behaviors of others, including trying to envision what it must be like to be in the position of the client and the client's family.

  - Nonjudgmental attitude – This is a display of acceptance that will encourage open, honest communication.

 View Media Supplement: Therapeutic and Nontherapeutic Communication (Video)

Nursing Process

- Assessment

  o Assess verbal and nonverbal communication needs.

  o Consider the client's developmental level and how communication should be altered during the assessment phase.

    ▪ Children

      ▫ Use simple, straightforward language.

      ▫ Be aware of own nonverbal messages, as children are sensitive to nonverbal communication.

      ▫ Enhance communication by being at the child's eye level.

      ▫ Incorporate play in interactions.

    ▪ Older Adult Clients

      ▫ Recognize that the client may require amplification.

      ▫ Minimize distractions, and face the client when speaking.

      ▫ Allow plenty of time for the client to respond.

      ▫ When impaired communication is assessed, ask for input from caregivers or family to determine the extent of the deficits and how best to communicate.

    ▪ Identify any cultural considerations that may impact communication.

- Planning

  o Minimize distractions.

  o Provide for privacy.

  o Identify mutually agreed-upon client outcomes.

  o Set priorities according to the client's needs.

  o Plan for adequate time for interventions.

- Implementation

  o Establish a trusting nurse-client relationship. The client feels more at ease during the implementation phase when a helping relationship has been established.

  o Provide empathetic responses and explanations to the client by using observations and providing hope, humor, and information.

 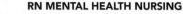

Effective Skills and Techniques

EFFECTIVE COMMUNICATION	INFLUENCE ON COMMUNICATION
Silence	Silence allows time for meaningful reflection.
Active listening	The nurse is able to hear, observe, and understand what the client communicates and to provide feedback.
Open-ended questions	This technique facilitates spontaneous responses and interactive discussion.
Clarifying techniques	This technique is used to determine if the message received was accurate: • Restating – uses the client's exact words. • Reflecting – directs the focus back to the client in order for the client to examine his feelings. • Paraphrasing – restates the client's feelings and thoughts for the client to confirm what has been communicated. • Exploring – allows the nurse to gather more information regarding important topics mentioned by the client.
Offering general leads, broad opening statements	This encourages the client to determine where the communication can start and to continue talking.
Showing acceptance and recognition	This technique acknowledges the nurse's interest and nonjudgmental attitude.
Focusing	This technique helps the client to concentrate on what is important.
Asking questions	Asking questions is a way to seek additional information.
Giving information	This technique provides details that the client may need for decision making.
Presenting reality	This technique is used to help the client focus on what is actually happening and to dispel delusions, hallucinations, or faulty beliefs.
Summarizing	Summarizing emphasizes important points and reviews what has been discussed.
Offering self	Use of this technique demonstrates a willingness to spend time with the client. Limited personal information may be shared, but the focus should return to the client as soon as possible. Relevant self-disclosure by the nurse allows the client to see that his experience is shared by others and understood.
Touch	If appropriate, touch communicates caring and may provide comfort to the client.

Barriers to Effective Communication

- Asking irrelevant personal questions
- Offering personal opinions
- Giving advice
- Giving false reassurance
- Minimizing feelings
- Changing the topic
- Asking "why" questions
- Offering value judgments
- Excessive questioning
- Responding approvingly or disapprovingly

Client Outcomes

- The client will verbalize concerns to the nurse.
- The client will request assistance from the nurse as appropriate.
- The client will communicate needs to the nurse.

CHAPTER 3: EFFECTIVE COMMUNICATION

(A) Application Exercises

1. Give two examples of how a nurse can use intrapersonal communication to enhance communication with a client.

2. Match the element of verbal communication with the appropriate example that could cause miscommunication to occur.

_____	Pacing	A. Use of medical jargon such as "decubitus ulcer"
_____	Connotative meaning	B. Charting that is written "client complains of" versus "client reports"
_____	Vocabulary	C. A client avoiding asking a nurse a question because the nurse is speaking rapidly and seems very busy
_____	Clarity	D. A nurse attempting to teach a client about her medications while the client is waiting for a phone call from her daughter
_____	Timing	E. A nurse distractingly using the phrase "um" repetitively in her communication

3. Which of the following is a barrier to therapeutic communication?

   A. Offering advice

   B. Reflecting meaning

   C. Listening attentively

   D. Giving information

4. Effective communication with clients and families is based on

   A. discussing topics with which the client feels comfortable.

   B. using silence to avoid unpleasant or difficult topics.

   C. attending to verbal and nonverbal behaviors.

   D. requesting the client to ask for feedback.

5. When a family asks a nurse for reassurance about a client's condition, which of the following is an appropriate response?

   A. "I think your son is getting better. What have you noticed?"

   B. "I'm sure everything will be okay. It just takes time to heal."

   C. "I'm not sure what's wrong. Have you asked the doctor about your concerns?"

   D. "I understand you're concerned. Let's discuss what concerns you specifically."

CHAPTER 3: EFFECTIVE COMMUNICATION

 Application Exercises Answer Key

1. Give two examples of how a nurse can use intrapersonal communication to enhance communication with a client.

> A nurse enters a client's room and sees that the client is crying. Using the technique of self-talk, the nurse asks herself, "I wonder why this client is so upset? Is he sad? Is he in pain? Does he have a social support system?" The nurse's assessment questions then stem from that intrapersonal communication. The nurse is using assessment skills to identify a potential problem, and she intervenes by asking the client pertinent questions to come to a more concrete answer.

> A client's condition is deteriorating, and the nurse must phone the primary care provider. Intrapersonally, the nurse goes through a "self-talk" discussion about what is to be said to the provider. This allows the nurse to be proactive and anticipate the provider's requests and/or questions. The nurse's intrapersonal communication enhances the interpersonal communication with the provider to best meet the needs of the client. The nurse is using "self-talk" to prepare for a future interpersonal communication encounter.

 NCLEX® Connection: Psychosocial Integrity, Therapeutic Communications

2. Match the element of verbal communication with the appropriate example that could cause miscommunication to occur.

__C__	Pacing	A. Use of medical jargon such as "decubitus ulcer"
__B__	Connotative meaning	B. Charting that is written "client complains of" versus "client reports"
__A__	Vocabulary	C. A client avoiding asking a nurse a question because the nurse is speaking rapidly and seems very busy
__E__	Clarity	D. A nurse attempting to teach a client about her medications while the client is waiting for a phone call from her daughter
__D__	Timing	E. A nurse distractingly using the phrase "um" repetitively in her communication

 NCLEX® Connection: Psychosocial Integrity, Therapeutic Communications

3. Which of the following is a barrier to therapeutic communication?

A. Offering advice

B. Reflecting meaning

C. Listening attentively

D. Giving information

Offering advice to a client should be avoided. Advice tends to interfere with the client's ability to make personal decisions and choices. The technique of reflection, on the other hand, encourages the client to make choices and is therapeutic. The skill of listening is an important therapeutic technique. Giving information informs the client of needed facts.

(N) NCLEX® Connection: Psychosocial Integrity, Therapeutic Communications

4. Effective communication with clients and families includes

A. discussing topics with which the client feels comfortable.

B. using silence to avoid unpleasant or difficult topics.

C. attending to verbal and nonverbal behaviors.

D. requesting the client to ask for feedback.

Attending to verbal and nonverbal behaviors is necessary for effective communication. In-depth conversations are not necessary for effective communication; often, very brief conversations are most effective. The purpose of effective silence is to allow the client time for reflection or to convey nonverbal support. Requiring the client to ask for feedback is not an effective technique.

(N) NCLEX® Connection: Psychosocial Integrity, Therapeutic Communications

5. When a family asks a nurse for reassurance about a client's condition, which of the following is an appropriate response?

A. "I think your son is getting better. What have you noticed?"

B. "I'm sure everything will be okay. It just takes time to heal."

C. "I'm not sure what's wrong. Have you asked the doctor about your concerns?"

D. "I understand you're concerned. Let's discuss what concerns you specifically."

A therapeutic response reflects upon, and accepts, the family's feelings, and it allows the members to clarify what they are feeling. Other responses interject the nurse's opinion and may cause the family to withhold their thoughts and feelings.

(N) NCLEX® Connection: Psychosocial Integrity, Therapeutic Communications

UNIT 1	FOUNDATIONS FOR MENTAL HEALTH NURSING
Chapter 4	Anxiety and Defense Mechanisms

Overview

- Stress can result from a change in one's environment that is threatening, causes challenges, or is perceived as damaging to that person's well-being. Stress causes anxiety.

- Dysfunctional behavior may occur when a defense mechanism is used as a response to anxiety.

- Individuals may use defense mechanisms as a way to manage conflict in response to anxiety. Defense mechanisms are reversible and can be adaptive, as well as maladaptive.

  - Adaptive use of defense mechanisms helps people to achieve their goals in acceptable ways. Defense mechanisms become maladaptive when they interfere with functioning, relationships, and orientation to reality.

  - It is important that the defense mechanism used is appropriate to the situation and that an individual uses a variety of defense mechanisms, rather than having the same reaction to every situation.

Defense Mechanisms

- Healthy defenses include altruism, sublimation, humor, and suppression.

- Intermediate defenses include repression, reaction formation, somatization, displacement, rationalization, and undoing.

- Immature defenses include projection, acting-out behaviors, dissociation, devaluation, idealization, splitting, passive aggression, and denial.

DEFENSE MECHANISM	DESCRIPTION	EXAMPLE
Altruism	Dealing with anxiety by reaching out to others	A nurse who lost a family member in a fire is a volunteer firefighter.
Sublimation	Dealing with unacceptable feelings or impulses by unconsciously substituting acceptable forms of expression	A person who has feelings of anger and hostility toward his work supervisor sublimates those feelings by working out vigorously at the gym during his lunch period.
Suppression	Voluntarily denying unpleasant thoughts and feelings	A person who has lost his job states he will worry about paying his bills next week.
Repression	Putting unacceptable ideas, thoughts, and emotions out of conscious awareness	A person who has a fear of the dentist's drill continually "forgets" his dental appointments.
Displacement	Shifting feelings related to an object, person, or situation to another less threatening object, person, or situation	A person who is angry about losing his job destroys his child's favorite toy.
Reaction formation	Overcompensating or demonstrating the opposite behavior of what is felt	A person who dislikes her sister's daughter offers to babysit so that her sister can go out of town.
Somatization	Developing a physical symptom in place of anxiety	A school-age child develops abdominal pain to avoid going to school, where he is being bullied.
Undoing	Performing an act to make up for prior behavior	An adolescent completes his chores without being prompted after having an argument with his parent.
Rationalization	Creating reasonable and acceptable explanations for unacceptable behavior	A young adult explains he had to drive home from a party after drinking alcohol because he had to feed his dog.
Passive aggression	Indirectly behaving aggressively but appearing to be compliant	A person's coworker agrees to take on one of her assignments but then does not meet the deadline.
Acting-out behaviors	Managing emotional conflicts through actions, rather than self-reflection	A preschool child is told to share her toys, so she throws the toys across the room.

DEFENSE MECHANISM	DESCRIPTION	EXAMPLE
Dissociation	Temporarily blocking memories and perceptions from consciousness	An adolescent witnesses a shooting and is unable to recall any details of the event.
Devaluation	Expressing negative thoughts of self or others	A person who is passed up for a promotion states that the job is not better than the one he currently has.
Idealization	Expressing extremely positive thoughts of self or others	A school-age boy boasts about his older brother and his accomplishments.
Splitting	Demonstrating an inability to reconcile negative and positive attributes of self or others	A client tells a nurse that she is the only one who cares about her, yet the following day, the same client refuses to talk to the nurse.
Projection	Blaming others for unacceptable thoughts and feelings	A young adult blames his substance abuse on his parents' refusal to buy him a new car.
Denial	Pretending the truth is not reality to manage the anxiety of acknowledging what is real	A parent who is informed that his son was killed in combat tells everyone he is coming home for the holidays.

Anxiety

- Anxiety is viewed on a continuum with increasing levels of anxiety leading to decreasing ability to function.

    o Normal – A healthy life force that is necessary for survival, normal anxiety motivates people to take action. For example, a potentially violent situation occurs on the mental health unit, and the nurse moves rapidly to defuse the situation. The anxiety experienced by the nurse during the situation helped him perform quickly and efficiently.

    o Acute (state) – This level of anxiety is precipitated by an imminent loss or change that threatens one's sense of security. For example, the sudden death of a loved one precipitates an acute state of anxiety.

    o Chronic (trait) – This level of anxiety is one that usually develops over time, often starting in childhood. The adult who experiences chronic anxiety may display that anxiety in physical symptoms, such as fatigue and frequent headaches.

- Assessment of a client's level of anxiety is basic to therapeutic intervention in any setting.

LEVELS OF ANXIETY	
Mild	<ul><li>Mild anxiety occurs in the normal experience of everyday living.</li><li>It increases one's ability to perceive reality.</li><li>There is an identifiable cause of the anxiety.</li><li>Other characteristics include a vague feeling of mild discomfort, impatience, and apprehension.</li></ul>
Moderate	<ul><li>Moderate anxiety occurs when mild anxiety escalates.</li><li>Slightly reduced perception and processing of information occurs, and selective inattention may occur.</li><li>Ability to think clearly is hampered, but learning and problem solving may still occur.</li><li>Other characteristics include concentration difficulties, tiredness, pacing, and increased heart rate and respiratory rate.</li><li>The client with this type of anxiety usually benefits from the direction of others.</li></ul>
Severe	<ul><li>Perceptual field is greatly reduced with distorted perceptions.</li><li>Learning and problem solving do not occur.</li><li>Other characteristics include confusion, feelings of impending doom, and aimless activity.</li><li>The client with severe anxiety usually is not able to take direction from others.</li></ul>
Panic-level	<ul><li>Panic-level anxiety is characterized by markedly disturbed behavior.</li><li>The client is not able to process what is occurring in the environment and may lose touch with reality.</li><li>The client experiences extreme fright and horror.</li><li>Other characteristics may include dysfunction in speech, inability to sleep, delusions, and hallucinations.</li></ul>

- Nursing interventions are implemented according to the level of anxiety that a client is experiencing.

NURSING INTERVENTIONS FOR THE CLIENT WITH MILD TO MODERATE LEVELS OF ANXIETY	
NURSING INTERVENTION	THERAPEUTIC INTENT
Use active listening to demonstrate willingness to help, and use specific communication techniques (open-ended questions, giving broad openings, exploring, and seeking clarification).	These interventions encourage the client to express feelings, develop trust, and identify the source of the anxiety.
Provide a calm presence, recognizing the client's distress.	This assists the client to focus and to begin to problem solve.
Evaluate past coping mechanisms.	This will assist the client to identify adaptive and nonadaptive coping mechanisms.
Explore alternatives to problem situations.	This intervention offers options for problem solving.
Encourage participation in activities, such as exercise that may temporarily relieve feelings of inner tension.	This provides the client with an outlet for pent-up tension, promotes endorphin release, and improves mental well-being.

NURSING INTERVENTIONS FOR THE CLIENT WITH SEVERE TO PANIC LEVELS OF ANXIETY	
NURSING INTERVENTION	THERAPEUTIC INTENT
Provide an environment that meets the physical and safety needs of the client. Remain with the client.	This intervention minimizes risk to the client. The client may be unaware of the need for basic things, such as fluids, food, and sleep.
Provide a quiet environment with minimal stimulation.	This helps to prevent intensification of the current level of anxiety.
Use medications and restraint, but only after less restrictive interventions have failed to decrease anxiety to safer levels.	Medications and/or restraint may be necessary to prevent harm to the client and providers.
Encourage gross motor activities, such as walking and other forms of exercise.	This provides the client with an outlet for pent-up tension, promotes endorphin release, and improves mental well-being.
Set limits by using firm, short, and simple statements. Repetition may be necessary.	Limit-setting can minimize risk to the client and providers. Clear, simple communication facilitates understanding.
Direct the client to acknowledge reality and focus on what is present in the environment.	Focusing on reality will assist with reducing the client's anxiety level.

CHAPTER 4: ANXIETY AND DEFENSE MECHANISMS

(A) Application Exercises

1. Match each defense mechanism below with the letter of the behavior that best illustrates it.

_____	Reaction formation	A. A child is punished by his mother and sent to his room, where he begins to kick and break apart a favorite toy.
_____	Denial	B. A woman who just lost her job, because she frequently was late for work, tells friends that it will be much better for her family if she stays home every day.
_____	Displacement	C. A woman who just lost an election to a hated rival declares, "She is such a sweet person, and I really like her!"
_____	Rationalization	D. A heavy smoker diagnosed with lung cancer says, "I'm coughing because I have that cold that everyone has been getting."
_____	Sublimation	E. A husband feels very angry with his wife, so he goes outside and begins energetically cutting up firewood with an axe.

2. A client in a primary care facility just learned that she must have a breast biopsy. As the nurse tries to give her information about the procedure, he notices that the client is perspiring and pale. Her breathing is rapid at about 28/min, and she says, "You'll have to excuse me; I don't quite understand what you're trying to tell me." The nurse should assess the client's anxiety as

   A. mild.

   B. moderate.

   C. severe.

   D. panic.

3. Which of the following is an appropriate nursing strategy when trying to give necessary information to a client with moderate anxiety?

   A. Reassure the client that everything will be okay.

   B. Encourage the client to talk about her feelings of anxiety.

   C. Ignore the client's anxiety so that she will not be embarrassed.

   D. Demonstrate a calm manner while using simple and clear language.

Scenario: A father enters the emergency department with his son, who has just been hit by a car. The father was supposed to be watching the 6 year old while the child's mother was out shopping; however, the child slipped out of the house and wandered into the street in front of his home. At the hospital, the child is immediately sent to surgery and is in critical condition. The father, who is still in the emergency department waiting room, is very distraught and is wailing loudly. He demonstrates an inability to be still, his hands are shaking, and he is frequently dropping his keys. "It should have been me," he moans. Others in the waiting room are starting to appear anxious and are complaining about the disturbance.

4. What level of anxiety is the father experiencing? What data support this description?

5. Identify three nursing interventions for the father.

CHAPTER 4: ANXIETY AND DEFENSE MECHANISMS

 Application Exercises Answer Key

1. Match each defense mechanism below with the letter of the behavior that best illustrates it.

C	Reaction formation	A. A child is punished by his mother and sent to his room, where he begins to kick and break apart a favorite toy.
D	Denial	B. A woman who just lost her job, because she frequently was late for work, tells friends that it will be much better for her family if she stays home every day.
A	Displacement	C. A woman who just lost an election to a hated rival declares, "She is such a sweet person, and I really like her!"
B	Rationalization	D. A heavy smoker diagnosed with lung cancer says, "I'm coughing because I have that cold that everyone has been getting."
E	Sublimation	E. A husband feels very angry with his wife, so he goes outside and begins energetically cutting up firewood with an axe.

NCLEX® Connection: Psychosocial Integrity, Mental Health Concepts

2. A client in a primary care facility just learned that she must have a breast biopsy. As the nurse tries to give her information about the procedure, he notices that the client is perspiring and pale. Her breathing is rapid at about 28/min, and she says, "You'll have to excuse me; I don't quite understand what you're trying to tell me." The nurse should assess the client's anxiety as

A. mild.

B. moderate.

C. severe.

D. panic.

Moderate anxiety decreases problem solving and may hamper one's ability to understand information. Vital signs may increase somewhat, and the person is visibly anxious. In mild anxiety, the person's ability to understand information may actually increase. Severe anxiety causes restlessness, decreased perception, and an inability to take direction. During a panic attack, the person is completely distracted, unable to function, and may lose touch with reality.

NCLEX® Connection: Psychosocial Integrity, Behavioral Interventions

3. Which of the following is an appropriate nursing strategy when trying to give necessary information to a client with moderate anxiety?

> A. Reassure the client that everything will be okay.
>
> B. Encourage the client to talk about her feelings of anxiety.
>
> C. Ignore the client's anxiety so that she will not be embarrassed.
>
> **D. Demonstrate a calm manner while using simple and clear language.**
>
> Giving information simply and calmly will help the client grasp essential facts. Offering false reassurance is a nontherapeutic intervention. Trying to make the client verbalize her feelings may offer more distraction. Ignoring the anxiety will not help the client manage the situation.

 NCLEX® Connection: Psychosocial Integrity, Behavioral Interventions

---

Scenario: A father enters the emergency department with his son, who has just been hit by a car. The father was supposed to be watching the 6 year old while the child's mother was out shopping; however, the child slipped out of the house and wandered into the street in front of his home. At the hospital, the child is immediately sent to surgery and is in critical condition. The father, who is still in the emergency department waiting room, is very distraught and is wailing loudly. He demonstrates an inability to be still, his hands are shaking, and he is frequently dropping his keys. "It should have been me," he moans. Others in the waiting room are starting to appear anxious and are complaining about the disturbance.

---

4. What level of anxiety is the father experiencing? What data support this description?

> **This man demonstrates severe anxiety. He has an extremely reduced attention span, psychomotor agitation, and he is yelling.**

 NCLEX® Connection: Psychosocial Integrity, Crisis Intervention

5. Identify three nursing interventions for the father.

> Appropriate interventions include: remaining with the father; providing a safe and secure environment; assessing for and responding to themes noted in his communication; using firm, short, simple statements to communicate with him; and addressing comfort and safety needs by providing fluids and nutrition.

 NCLEX® Connection: Psychosocial Integrity, Crisis Intervention

UNIT 1	FOUNDATIONS FOR MENTAL HEALTH NURSING
Chapter 5	Creating and Maintaining a Therapeutic and Safe Environment

Overview

- Therapeutic encounters can occur in any nursing setting if a nurse is sensitive to a client's needs and uses effective communication skills.

- The therapeutic nurse-client relationship is foundational to mental health nursing care.

- The therapeutic nurse-client relationship differs from social and intimate relationships. A therapeutic nurse-client relationship is:

  o Purposeful and goal-directed

  o Well-defined with clear boundaries

  o Structured to meet the client's needs

  o Characterized by an interpersonal process that is safe, confidential, reliable, and consistent

- Milieu therapy creates an environment that is supportive, therapeutic and safe.

  o Milieu therapy began as an effort to provide an environment conducive to the treatment of children who were mentally ill.

  o Management of the milieu refers to the management of the total environment of the mental health unit in order to provide the least amount of stress, while promoting the greatest benefit for all the clients.

  o The goal is that while the client is in this therapeutic environment, he will learn the tools necessary to cope adaptively, interact more effectively and appropriately, and strengthen relationship skills. Hopefully, the client will use these tools in all other aspects of his life.

  o The nurse, as manager of care, is responsible for structuring and/or implementing aspects of the therapeutic milieu within the mental health facility.

  o One structure of the therapeutic milieu is regular community meetings, which include both the clients and the nursing staff.

The Therapeutic Nurse-Client Relationship

- Roles of the Nurse

  o Consistently focus on the client's ideas, experiences, and feelings.

  o Identify and explore the client's needs and problems.

  o Discuss problem-solving alternatives with the client.

- o   Help to develop the client's strengths and new coping skills.

- o   Encourage positive behavior change in the client.

- o   Assist the client to develop a sense of autonomy and self-reliance.

- o   Portray genuineness, empathy, and a positive regard toward the client.

- •   Benefits of the Therapeutic Relationship

    - o   Therapeutic relationships contribute to the well-being of those who are seriously mentally ill, as well as other clients, although the treatment goals will be individualized.

    - o   These relationships take time to establish, but even time-limited therapeutic encounters can have positive outcomes.

    - o   Therapeutic relationships have a positive impact on the success of treatment.

- •   Supervision by peers or the clinical team enhances the nurse's ability to examine her own thoughts and feelings, maintain boundaries, and continue to learn from nurse-client relationships.

FACTORS THAT POSITIVELY AFFECT THE DEVELOPMENT OF THE THERAPEUTIC RELATIONSHIP	
NURSE FACTORS	CLIENT FACTORS
• Consistent approach to interaction • Adjustment of pace to client's needs • Attentive listening • Positive initial impressions • Comfort level during the relationship • Self-awareness of own thoughts and feelings • Consistent availability	• Trusting attitude • Willingness to talk • Active participation • Consistent availability

PHASES AND TASKS OF A THERAPEUTIC RELATIONSHIP		
PHASE	NURSE	CLIENT
Orientation	• Introduce self to the client and state purpose. • Set the contract: meeting time, place, frequency, duration, and date of termination. • Discuss confidentiality. • Build trust by establishing expectations and boundaries. • Set goals with the client. • Explore the client's ideas, issues, and needs. • Explore the meaning of testing behaviors. • Enforce limits on testing or other inappropriate behaviors.	• Meet with the nurse. • Agree to the contract. • Understand the limits of confidentiality. • Understand the expectations and limits of the relationship. • Participate in setting goals. • Begin to explore own thoughts, experiences, and feelings. • Explore the meaning of own behaviors.

PHASES AND TASKS OF A THERAPEUTIC RELATIONSHIP		
PHASE	NURSE	CLIENT
Working	• Maintain relationship according to the contract. • Perform ongoing assessment to plan and evaluate therapeutic measures. • Facilitate the client's expression of needs and issues. • Encourage the client to problem solve. • Promote the client's self-esteem. • Foster positive behavioral change. • Explore and deal with resistance and other defense mechanisms. • Recognize transference and countertransference issues. • Reassess the client's problems and goals, and revise plans as necessary. • Support the client's adaptive alternatives and use of new coping skills. • Remind the client about the date of termination.	• Explore problematic areas of life. • Reconsider usual coping behaviors. • Examine own worldview and self-concept. • Describe major conflicts and various defenses. • Experience intense feelings, and learn to cope with anxiety reactions. • Test new behaviors. • Begin to develop awareness of transference situations. • Try alternative solutions.
Termination	• Provide opportunity for the client to discuss thoughts and feelings about termination and loss. • Discuss the client's previous experience with separations and loss. • Elicit the client's feelings about the therapeutic work in the nurse-client relationship. • Summarize goals and achievements. • Review memories of work in the sessions. • Express own feelings about sessions to validate the experience with the client. • Discuss ways for the client to incorporate new healthy behaviors into life. • Maintain limits of final termination.	• Discuss thoughts and feelings about termination. • Examine previous separation and loss experiences. • Explore the meaning of the therapeutic relationship. • Review goals and achievements. • Discuss plans to continue new behaviors. • Express any feelings of loss related to termination. • Make plans for the future. • Accept termination as final.

- Boundaries of the Therapeutic Relationship

  ○ Boundaries must be established in order to maintain a safe and professional nurse-client relationship.

  ○ Blurred boundaries occur if the relationship begins to meet the needs of the nurse rather than those of the client, or if the relationship becomes social rather than therapeutic.

  ○ The nurse must work to maintain a consistent level of involvement with the client, to reflect on boundary issues frequently, and to maintain awareness of how behaviors can be perceived by others (clients, family members, other health team members).

TRANSFERENCE AND COUNTERTRANSFERENCE			
BEHAVIOR	DESCRIPTION	EXAMPLE	NURSING IMPLICATIONS
Transference	Transference occurs when the client views a member of the health care team as having characteristics of another person who has been significant to the client's personal life.	A client may see a nurse as being like his mother, and thus may demonstrate some of the same behaviors with the nurse as he demonstrated with his mother.	A nurse should be aware that transference by a client is more likely to occur with a person in authority.
Countertransference	Countertransference occurs when a health care team member displaces characteristics of people in her past onto a client.	A nurse may feel defensive and angry with a client for no apparent reason if the client reminds her of a friend who often elicited those feelings.	A nurse should be aware that clients who induce very strong personal feelings may become objects of countertransference.

CHARACTERISTICS OF THE THERAPEUTIC MILIEU	
Physical Setting	• Unit should be clean and orderly. • Color scheme and overall design should be appropriate for the client's age. • The setting should include comfortable furniture placed so that it promotes interaction, solitary spaces for reading and thinking alone, comfortable places conducive to meals, and quiet areas for sleeping. • Materials used for such features as floors should be attractive, easy to clean, and safe. • Traffic-flow considerations should be conducive to client and staff movement.

CHARACTERISTICS OF THE THERAPEUTIC MILIEU	
Health Care Team Member Responsibilities	• Promote independence for self-care and individual growth in clients. • Treat clients as individuals. • Allow choices for clients within the daily routine and within individual treatment plans. • Apply rules of fair treatment for all clients. • Model good social behavior for clients, such as respect for the rights of others. • Work cooperatively as a team to provide care. • Maintain boundaries with clients. • Maintain a professional appearance and demeanor. • Promote safe and satisfying peer interactions among the clients. • Practice open communication techniques with health team members and clients. • Promote feelings of self-worth and hope for the future.
Emotional climate	• Clients should feel safe from harm (self-harm, as well as harm from disruptive behaviors of other clients). • Clients should feel cared for and accepted by the staff and others.

- Physical Safety

  o The nurses' station and other areas should be placed to allow for easy observation of clients by staff and access to staff by clients.

  o Special safety features, such as bathroom bars and wheelchair accessibility for clients who are disabled, should be addressed.

  o Set up the following provisions to prevent client self-harm or harm by others:

    ▪ No access to sharp or otherwise harmful objects

    ▪ Restriction of client access to restricted or locked areas

    ▪ Monitoring of visitors

    ▪ Restriction of alcohol and illegal drug access or use

    ▪ Restriction of sexual activity among clients

    ▪ Deterrence of elopement from facility

    ▪ Rapid de-escalation of disruptive and potentially violent behaviors through planned interventions by trained staff

  o Seclusion rooms and restraints should be set up for safety and used only after all less restrictive measures have been exhausted. When used, facility policies and procedures must be followed.

  o Plan for safe access to recreational areas, occupational therapy, and meeting rooms.

- ○ Teach fire, evacuation, and other safety rules to all staff.

  - ▪ Have clear plans for keeping clients and staff safe in emergencies.

  - ▪ Maintain staff skills, such as cardiopulmonary resuscitation.

- ○ Considerations of room assignments on a 24-hr inpatient unit should include:

  - ▪ Personalities of each roommate

  - ▪ The likelihood of nighttime disruptions for a roommate if one client has difficulty sleeping

  - ▪ Medical diagnoses, such as how two clients with severe paranoia might interact with each other

- ○ Activities within the therapeutic milieu are structured and include time for the following:

  - ▪ Community meetings

    - □ The community meeting on the mental health unit should enhance the emotional climate of the therapeutic milieu by promoting:

      - ▸ Interaction and communication between staff and clients

      - ▸ Decision-making skills of clients

      - ▸ A feeling of self-worth among clients

      - ▸ Discussions of common unit objectives, such as encouraging clients to meet treatment goals, and plan for discharge

      - ▸ Discussion of issues of concern to all members of the unit, including common problems, future activities, and the introduction of new clients to the unit

      - ▸ Meetings may be structured so that they are client-led with decisions made by the group as a whole.

  - ▪ Individual therapy – scheduled sessions with a mental health provider to address specific mental health concerns, such as depression

  - ▪ Group therapy – scheduled sessions for a group of clients to address common mental health issues, such as substance abuse

  - ▪ Psychoeducational groups – based on a client's level of functioning and personal needs, such as medication side effect

  - ▪ Recreational activities, such as a game or a community outing

  - ▪ Unstructured, flexible time that includes opportunities for the nurse and other staff to observe clients as they interact spontaneously within the milieu

CHAPTER 5: CREATING AND MAINTAINING A THERAPEUTIC AND SAFE ENVIRONMENT

(A) Application Exercises

1. A client says to a nurse, "Why should I talk to you? Everybody knows talking doesn't help!" Which of the following is an appropriate response by the nurse?

    A. "Why don't you let me be the judge of that?"

    B. "Your doctor said talking is part of your therapy."

    C. "Why do you think that talking won't help?"

    D. "I'm here to talk with you about your concerns."

2. A nurse is caring for a client who follows her around the unit and tries to engage her in conversation, after the nurse has set up a specific time for interaction. The client's behavior is an example of which of the following?

    A. Stalking

    B. Close rapport

    C. Inability to accept limits

    D. Sign of loneliness

3. Which of the following are characteristics of the nurse-client relationship? (Select all that apply.)

    _____ The needs of both participants are met.

    _____ An emotional commitment exists between the participants.

    _____ It is goal-directed.

    _____ Behavioral change is encouraged.

4. The termination phase of the nurse-client relationship focuses on which of the following?

    A. Discussing ways to use new behaviors

    B. Practicing new problem-solving skills

    C. Developing goals

    D. Experiencing intense feelings

5. A nurse is orienting a new client to an inpatient mental health unit. When explaining the unit's community meetings, the nurse should state which of the following to the client?

    A. "You and a group of other clients will meet to discuss your medication and treatment plans."

    B. "I never know what goes on at a community meeting, because the clients control the agenda."

    C. "You and the other clients will meet with staff to discuss activities, problems, and other things of interest to all."

    D. "You will meet alone with your therapist to discuss your treatment plan and problems you are having."

6. A client who is newly admitted to the acute care mental health unit has a DSM-IV-TR Axis I diagnosis of paranoid schizophrenia. The client is very frightened and delusional. During the client's first few days of treatment, which of the following aspects of the therapeutic milieu is most important?

    A. Socialization with other clients

    B. Structured activities with staff

    C. Recreational therapy in the community

    D. Communication in group therapy

CHAPTER 5: CREATING AND MAINTAINING A THERAPEUTIC AND SAFE ENVIRONMENT

 Application Exercises Answer Key

1. A client says to a nurse, "Why should I talk to you? Everybody knows talking doesn't help!" Which of the following is an appropriate response by the nurse?

    A. "Why don't you let me be the judge of that?"

    B. "Your doctor said talking is part of your therapy."

    C. "Why do you think that talking won't help?"

    D. "I'm here to talk with you about your concerns."

An appropriate response is a broad opening that focuses on the client's feelings and needs. Option A minimizes the client's ability to make decisions and is obstructive to open expression of feelings. Option B changes the focus of the interview to the primary care provider's orders. Option C implies criticism of the client's response, which could possibly make the client defensive. It is important to avoid minimizing the client's feelings, focusing attention away from the client, or implying criticism of the client's response.

 NCLEX® Connection: Psychosocial Integrity, Therapeutic Environment

2. A nurse is caring for a client who follows her around the unit and tries to engage her in conversation, after the nurse has set up a specific time for interaction. The client's behavior is an example of which of the following?

    A. Stalking

    B. Close rapport

    C. Inability to accept limits

    D. Sign of loneliness

Limits must be set so that one client will not monopolize a nurse's time. This may be a boundary issue for the client and nurse. There is no evidence that this is a stalking behavior, a sign of close rapport with the nurse, or that the client is lonely.

 NCLEX® Connection: Psychosocial Integrity, Therapeutic Environment

3. Which of the following are characteristics of the nurse-client relationship? (Select all that apply.)

    _____ The needs of both participants are met.

    _____ An emotional commitment exists between the participants.

    __**X**__ **It is goal-directed.**

    __**X**__ **Behavioral change is encouraged.**

In order for a nurse-client relationship to be therapeutic and beneficial for the client, there must be clear boundaries; there must be clearly identified goals toward which the client is working; and the nurse must encourage behavioral change to improve the client's mental health. The needs of both participants may be met in a social relationship, and an emotional commitment exists between participants in an intimate relationship.

 NCLEX® Connection: Psychosocial Integrity, Therapeutic Environment

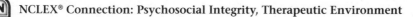

4. The termination phase of the nurse-client relationship focuses on which of the following?

   A. Discussing ways to use new behaviors

   B. Practicing new problem-solving skills

   C. Developing goals

   D. Experiencing intense feelings

   During the termination phase, the nurse and the client discuss ways that the client can use newly learned behaviors. Practicing new problem-solving skills and experiencing intense feelings usually takes place during the working phase. Developing goals should take place in the orientation phase.

   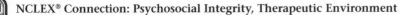 NCLEX® Connection: Psychosocial Integrity, Therapeutic Environment

5. A nurse is orienting a new client to an inpatient mental health unit. When explaining the unit's community meetings, the nurse should state which of the following to the client?

   A. "You and a group of other clients will meet to discuss your medication and treatment plans."

   B. "I never know what goes on at a community meeting, because the clients control the agenda."

   C. "You and the other clients will meet with staff to discuss activities, problems, and other things of interest to all."

   D. "You will meet alone with your therapist to discuss your treatment plan and problems you are having."

   Community meetings include both staff and clients on a unit. Any topic of interest to the entire group may be discussed, including problems, future activities, and meeting new clients.

   NCLEX® Connection: Psychosocial Integrity, Therapeutic Environment

6. A client who is newly admitted to the acute care mental health unit has a DSM-IV-TR Axis I diagnosis of paranoid schizophrenia. The client is very frightened and delusional. During the client's first few days of treatment, which of the following aspects of the therapeutic milieu is most important?

   A. Socialization with other clients

   B. Structured activities with staff

   C. Recreational therapy in the community

   D. Communication in group therapy

   The greatest risk to this client is injury to self and others. Structured activities are the most effective ways to provide a safe environment for the client, staff, and other clients. Socialization, recreational therapy, and attendance at group therapy are all important aspects of the therapeutic milieu, but they are not the most important for this client.

   NCLEX® Connection: Psychosocial Integrity, Therapeutic Environment

Overview

- Acute Care Settings for Mental Health Care

  - This setting provides intensive treatment and supervision in locked units for clients with severe mental illness.

  - Care in these facilities helps stabilize mental illness symptoms and promotes the client's return to the community.

  - Staff is made up of an interdisciplinary team with management provided by nurses.

  - Facilities may be privately owned, with payment provided by private funds or insurance.

  - Facilities may also be state owned, with much of the funding provided for indigent clients. State-run facilities also often provide full-time acute care for forensic clients (those in a correctional setting) with severe mental illness.

  - Case management programs assist with client transition to a community setting after discharge from the acute care facility.

- Community Settings for Mental Health Care

  - Primary care is provided in community-based settings, which include clinics, schools and daycare centers, partial hospitalization programs, drug and alcohol treatment facilities, forensic settings, psychosocial rehabilitation programs, telephone crisis counseling centers, and home health care.

  - Nurses working in community care programs help to stabilize or improve a client's mental functioning within a community and teach, support, and make referrals in order to promote positive social activities.

  - Nursing interventions in community settings provide for primary treatment and primary, secondary, and tertiary prevention of mental illness.

- In all settings, nurses are advocates for clients with mental illness. Referral of clients and their families to organizations and agencies that provide additional resources can provide significant support to individuals. For example, the National Alliance on Mental Illness (NAMI), is a grassroots organization with the goals of improving the quality of life for persons with mental illness and for providing research to better treat or eradicate mental illness. For more information, go to http://www.nami.org/.

History of Mental Health Care in the United States

- Most clients with severe mental illness were treated solely in acute care inpatient facilities before the middle of the twentieth century.

- Congress passed a series of acts in 1946, 1955, and 1963 in response to the appalling condition of facilities for the mentally ill. This began a trend to deinstitutionalize mental health care.

- Clients who had lived in acute care mental health facilities for many years were discharged into the community at a time when community mental health facilities were often unprepared to deal with this influx.

- The concept of the case manager was introduced around 1970 to meet the individual needs of a client in a mental health setting.

- Managed care through Health Maintenance Organizations (HMOs), Preferred Provider Organizations (PPOs), and others began limiting hospital stays for clients in a general medical setting starting around 1980.

  - Managed Behavioral Healthcare Organizations (MBHOs) were later developed to coordinate care and limit stays in acute care facilities for clients needing mental health care.

  - This began the trend to develop a continuum of acute care facilities, as well as community mental health facilities to provide for all levels of behavioral health care needs.

  - Complete and accurate documentation of client needs and progress by nurses and other health care providers is necessary to assure quality client care for each individual.

- Factors that will affect the future of mental health care include:

  - An increase in the aging population

  - An increase in cultural diversity within the United States

  - The expansion of technology, which may provide new settings for client care, as well as new ways to treat mental illness more effectively

Client Care In Acute Mental Health Care Settings

- Criteria to justify admission to an acute care facility include:

  - A clear risk of the client's danger to self or others

  - The failure of community-based treatment

  - A dangerous decline in the mental health status of a client undergoing long-term treatment

  - A client having a medical need in addition to a mental illness

- Goals of acute mental health treatment include:

  ○ Prevention of the client harming self or others

  ○ Stabilizing mental health crises

  ○ Return of clients who are severally ill to some type of community care

- Interdisciplinary team members in acute care include nurses, mental health technicians (who perform duties similar to assistive personnel in other health care facilities), psychologists, psychiatrists, other general health care providers, social workers, counselors, occupational and other specialty therapists, and pharmacists.

  ○ The interdisciplinary team has the primary responsibility of planning and monitoring individualized treatment plans or clinical pathways of care, depending on the philosophy and policy of the facility.

  ○ Plans for discharge to home or to a community facility/agency begin from the time of admission and continue with the implementation of the initial treatment plan or clinical pathway.

  ○ Nurses in acute care mental health facilities use the nursing process, as well as a holistic approach, to provide care. Nursing roles include:

    ▪ Overall management of the unit, including client activities and therapeutic milieu

    ▪ Assuring safe administration and monitoring of all client medications

    ▪ Implementation of individual client treatment plans, including client teaching

    ▪ Documentation of the nursing process for each client

    ▪ Managing crises as they arise

Client Care In Community Health Settings

- Nurses are mainly responsible for linking acute care facilities with community care facilities.

- Intensive outpatient programs promote community reintegration for clients.

- Three levels of prevention are utilized by nurses when implementing community care interventions/teaching.

LEVEL OF PREVENTION	EXAMPLES OF INTERVENTIONS
Primary prevention promotes health and prevents mental health problems from occurring.	The nurse leads a group for parents of toddlers, discussing normal toddler behavior and ways to promote healthy development.
Secondary prevention focuses on early detection of mental illness.	The nurse screens the parents of children who have developmental disorders.
Tertiary prevention focuses on rehabilitation and prevention of further problems in clients previously diagnosed.	The nurse leads a support group for clients who have completed a chemical dependency program.

- Community-based mental health programs are a continuum of mental health agencies with varying treatment intensity levels to allow clients to remain safe in the least restrictive environment possible.

  ○ Community-based mental health programs include:

COMMUNITY SETTING	GENERAL FUNCTION AND EXAMPLES OF CARE
Partial hospitalization programs	• These programs provide intense short-term treatment for clients who are well enough to go home every night and who have a responsible person at home to provide support and a safe environment. • Certain detoxification programs are a specialized form of partial hospitalization for the client who requires medical supervision, stress management, addiction counseling, and relapse prevention.
Assertive community treatment (ACT)	• This includes nontraditional case management and treatment by an interdisciplinary team for a caseload of clients with severe mental illness who are noncompliant with traditional treatment. • ACT helps to reduce reoccurrences of hospitalizations and provides crisis intervention, assistance with independent living, and information regarding resources for necessary support services.
Community mental health centers	These facilities provide a variety of services for a wide range of community clients, including: • Educational groups • Medication dispensing programs • Individual counseling programs
Psychosocial rehabilitation programs	These programs provide a structured range of programs for clients in a mental health setting, including: • Residential services • Day programs for older adults for whom care is provided
Home care	Home care provides mental health assessment, interventions, and family support in the client's own home. This is implemented most often for children, older adults, and clients with medical conditions.

Roles of Nurses In Diverse Mental Health Practice Settings

REGISTERED NURSE	ADVANCED PRACTICE NURSE
Educational preparation: diploma, associate degree, or baccalaureate degree in nursing, with additional on-the-job training and continuing education in mental health care	Educational preparation: advanced nursing degree in behavioral health (master's degree, doctorate, nurse practitioner, or clinical nurse specialist)
May work in either an acute care or community-based facility	May work independently, often supervising individuals or groups in either an acute care or community-based setting
Functions within a facility using the nursing process to provide care and treatment, such as medication	May have prescription privileges and is able to independently recommend interventions
Manages care for a group of clients within a unit of the facility	May manage and administrate care for an entire facility

CHAPTER 6: DIVERSE PRACTICE SETTINGS

 Application Exercises

1. A staff nurse provides direct client care in an acute care mental health facility. Which of the following aspects of care should the nurse perform?

   A. Physical care

   B. Vocational guidance

   C. Art therapy

   D. Mental status assessment

2. Four clients have been living alone in studio apartments with regular visits from a nurse case worker. Which of the following clients should the nurse plan to visit first?

   A. A client who recently burned her arm while using a hot iron at home

   B. A client who requests that her antipsychotic medication be changed due to some new side effects

   C. A client who says he is hearing a voice that tells him he is not worthy of living anymore

   D. A client who tells the nurse he experienced symptoms of severe anxiety before and during a job interview

3. A nurse is teaching healthy coping skills to older adult clients who have been hospitalized previously for severe depression and are now in a residential care facility. This is an example of which of the following?

   A. Primary prevention

   B. Secondary prevention

   C. Tertiary prevention

   D. Mental status examination

4. Which of the following clients should a nurse consider for referral to an assertive community treatment (ACT) group?

   A. A client in an acute care mental health facility who has fallen several times while running down the hallway

   B. A client who lives at home and keeps "forgetting" to come in for his monthly antipsychotic injection for schizophrenia

   C. A client in a day treatment program who says he is becoming more anxious during group therapy

   D. A client in a weekly grief support group who says she still misses her deceased husband who has been dead for 3 months

5. A client who has a severe mental illness will soon be ready for discharge from an acute mental health facility, but he still requires supervision much of the time. His wife works all day but is home by late afternoon. Which of the following should the nurse suggest as appropriate follow-up care?

    A. Receiving daily care from a home health aide

    B. Having a weekly visit from a nurse case worker

    C. Attending a partial hospitalization program

    D. Visiting a community mental health center on a daily basis

CHAPTER 6: DIVERSE PRACTICE SETTINGS

 Application Exercises Answer Key

1. A staff nurse provides direct client care in an acute care mental health facility. Which of the following aspects of care should the nurse perform?

    A. Physical care

    B. Vocational guidance

    C. Art therapy

    D. Mental status assessment

    One of many nursing responsibilities in an acute care mental health facility is to assess a client's mental status. A mental health technician or assistive personnel can perform physical care. The social worker provides care, such as vocational guidance. An occupational or specialized activity therapist would provide art therapy.

 NCLEX® Connection: Psychosocial Integrity, Behavioral Interventions

2. Four clients have been living alone in studio apartments with regular visits from a nurse case worker. Which of the following clients should the nurse plan to visit first?

    A. A client who recently burned her arm while using a hot iron at home

    B. A client who requests that her antipsychotic medication be changed due to some new side effects

    C. A client who says he is hearing a voice that tells him he is not worthy of living anymore

    D. A client who tells the nurse he experienced symptoms of severe anxiety before and during a job interview

    A client who hears a voice telling him he is not worthy of living is at greatest risk for self-harm. The other clients have needs that should be met but are not as high a priority as the client at risk for self-injury.

 NCLEX® Connection: Psychosocial Integrity, Crisis Intervention

3. A nurse is working on promotion of healthy coping skills with older adult clients who had all previously been hospitalized for severe depression and are now in a residential care facility. This is an example of which of the following?

    A. Primary prevention

    B. Secondary prevention

    C. Tertiary prevention

    D. Mental status examination

    Tertiary prevention deals with preventing further problems in clients already diagnosed with mental illness. Primary prevention deals with preventing the initial onset of a mental health problem. Secondary prevention deals with early detection of disease. Mental status examination is a tool that the nurse could use to assess a client's problem, but it is not a type of prevention.

 NCLEX® Connection: Psychosocial Integrity, Therapeutic Environment

4. Which of the following clients should a nurse consider for referral to an assertive community treatment (ACT) group?

A. A client in an acute care mental health facility who has fallen several times while running down the hallway

B. A client who lives at home and keeps "forgetting" to come in for his monthly antipsychotic injection for schizophrenia

C. A client in a day treatment program who says he is becoming more anxious during group therapy

D. A client in a weekly grief support group who says she still misses her deceased husband who has been dead for 3 months

An ACT group works with clients who are noncompliant with traditional therapy, such as the client in a home setting who keeps "forgetting" his injection. The client in acute care who has been running and falling should be helped by the treatment team on her unit. The client with anxiety might be referred to his counselor or mental health provider. The client who is grieving for her husband who died 3 months ago is currently involved in an appropriate intervention.

(N) NCLEX® Connection: Psychosocial Integrity, Therapeutic Environment

5. A client who has a severe mental illness will soon be ready for discharge from an acute mental health facility, but he still requires supervision much of the time. His wife works all day but is home by late afternoon. Which of the following should the nurse suggest as appropriate follow-up care?

A. Receiving daily care from a home health aide

B. Having a weekly visit from a nurse case worker

C. Attending a partial hospitalization program

D. Visiting a community mental health center on a daily basis

A partial hospitalization program can provide treatment during the day while allowing the client to spend nights at home, as long as a responsible family member is present. Daily care provided by a home health aide, a weekly visit from a nurse case worker, and daily visits to a community health center will not provide adequate care and supervision for this client.

(N) NCLEX® Connection: Psychosocial Integrity, Therapeutic Environment

UNIT 2: TRADITIONAL NONPHARMACOLOGICAL THERAPIES

- Psychoanalysis, Psychotherapy, and Behavioral Therapies
- Group and Family Therapy
- Stress Management
- Electroconvulsive Therapy

NCLEX® CONNECTIONS

When reviewing the chapters in this unit, keep in mind the relevant sections of the NCLEX® outline, in particular:

CLIENT NEEDS: PSYCHOSOCIAL INTEGRITY

Relevant topics/tasks include:
- Behavioral Interventions
  - Participate in group sessions.
- Family Dynamics
  - Encourage client participation in group/family therapy.
- Mental Health Concepts
  - Recognize the client's use of defense mechanisms.
- Stress Management
  - Implement measures to reduce environmental stressors.
- Support Systems
  - Assist family to plan care for the client with impaired cognition.

CLIENT NEEDS: REDUCTION OF RISK POTENTIAL

Relevant topics/tasks include:
- Potential for Complications of Diagnostic Tests/Treatments/Procedures
  - Provide care for the client undergoing electroconvulsive therapy.

UNIT 2	TRADITIONAL NONPHARMACOLOGICAL THERAPIES
Chapter 7	Psychoanalysis, Psychotherapy, and Behavioral Therapies

Overview

- Psychoanalysis, psychotherapy, and behavioral therapies are approaches to addressing mental health issues using various methods and theoretical bases.

- Nurses working in mental health settings should be familiar with the methods employed among these approaches and how they are applied in practice.

Psychoanalysis

- Classical psychoanalysis is a therapeutic process of assessing unconscious thoughts and feelings, and resolving conflict through talking to a psychoanalyst for many sessions and over months to years.

  ○ Due to the length of psychoanalytic therapy and health insurance constraints, classical psychoanalysis is less likely to be used as the sole therapy of choice.

  ○ Psychoanalysis was first developed by Sigmund Freud in order to resolve internal conflicts which, Freud contended, always occur from early childhood experiences.

  ○ Past relationships are a common focus for therapy.

- Therapeutic tools include:

  ○ Free association, which is the spontaneous, uncensored verbalization of whatever comes to a client's mind

  ○ Dream analysis and interpretation

  ○ Transference, which includes feelings that the client has developed toward the therapist related to similar feelings toward significant persons in the client's early childhood

  ○ Use of defense mechanisms

- Psychotherapy involves more verbal therapist-to-client interaction than classic psychoanalysis.

  ○ A trusting relationship is developed between the client and the therapist in order to explore the client's problems.

  ○ Psychodynamic psychotherapy employs the same tools as psychoanalysis but is oriented more to the client's present state rather than his early life.

- ○ Interpersonal psychotherapy (IPT) is used for clients with specific problems. It can improve interpersonal relationships, communication, role-relationship, and bereavement.

- ○ Cognitive therapy is based on the cognitive model, which focuses on individual thoughts and behaviors to solve current problems. It is used to treat depression, anxiety, eating disorders, and other issues that can be improved by changing a client's attitude toward life experiences.

- ○ Behavioral Therapy

  - ■ In protest of Freud's psychoanalytic theory, behavioral theorists such as Ivan Pavlov, John B. Watson, and B.F. Skinner felt that changing behavior was the key to treating problems such as anxiety and depression.

  - ■ Behavioral therapy is based on the theory that behavior is learned and has consequences. Abnormal behavior results from an attempt to avoid painful feelings. Changing abnormal or maladaptive behavior can occur without the need for insight into the underlying cause of the behavior.

  - ■ Behavioral therapies teach clients ways to decrease anxiety or avoidant behavior and give clients an opportunity to practice techniques.

  - ■ Behavioral therapy has been used successfully to treat clients with phobias, addictions, and other issues.

- ○ Cognitive-behavioral therapy uses both a cognitive and behavioral approach to assist a client with anxiety management.

Use of Cognitive Therapy

- • Cognitive Reframing

  - ○ Anxiety can be decreased by changing cognitive distortions. Cognitive reframing assists clients to identify negative thoughts that produce anxiety, examine the cause, and develop supportive ideas that replace negative self-talk. For example, a client who is depressed may say he is "a bad person" who has "never done anything good" in his life. Through therapy, this client may change his thinking to realize that he may have made some bad choices, but that he is not "a bad person."

    - ■ Priority restructuring – assists clients to identify what should be given priority, such as devoting energy to pleasurable activities.

    - ■ Journal keeping – helps clients write down stressful thoughts and has a positive effect on well-being

    - ■ Assertiveness training – teaches clients to express feelings, and solve problems in a nonaggressive manner.

    - ■ Monitoring thoughts – helps clients to be aware of negative thinking.

Types and Uses of Behavioral Therapy

TYPE	DEFINITION	USE IN MENTAL HEALTH NURSING
Modeling	The therapist or others serve as role models for the client, who learns improved behavior by imitation.	Modeling has been used in the acute care milieu to help clients improve interpersonal skills. The therapist demonstrates appropriate behavior in a stressful situation with the goal of having the client imitate the behavior.
Operant conditioning	Positive rewards are given for positive behavior (positive reinforcement).	As an example: tokens are given to clients for good behavior, and they can be exchanged by the client for a privilege or other items.
Systematic desensitization	This therapy is the planned, progressive, or graduated exposure to anxiety-provoking stimuli in real-life situations, or by imagining events that cause anxiety. During this exposure, the anxiety response is suppressed through the use of relaxation techniques.	Systematic desensitization begins with the client mastering relaxation techniques. Then the client is exposed to increasing levels of the anxiety-producing stimulus (either imagined or real) and uses relaxation to overcome anxiety. The client is then able to tolerate a greater and greater level of the stimulus until anxiety no longer interferes with functioning.
Aversion therapy	A maladaptive behavior is paired with a punishment or unpleasant stimuli to change the behavior.	A therapist or treatment team may use unpleasant stimuli, such as bitter taste or mild electric shock, as punishment for behaviors such as alcoholism, violence, self-mutilation, and thumb sucking.
Meditation, guided imagery, diaphragmatic breathing, muscle relaxation, and biofeedback	Various techniques are used to control pain, tension, and anxiety.	As an example, a nurse can teach diaphragmatic breathing to a client having a panic attack, or to a female client in labor.

- Other techniques include:

  ○ Flooding: exposing a client, while accompanied by a therapist, to a great deal of an undesirable stimulus in an attempt to turn off the anxiety response.

  ○ Response prevention: preventing a client from performing a compulsive behavior with the intent that anxiety will be diminished

  ○ Thought stopping: Teaching a client, when negative thoughts or compulsive behaviors arise, to say or shout, "stop," and substitute a positive thought. The goal over time is for the client to use the command silently.

CHAPTER 7: PSYCHOANALYSIS, PSYCHOTHERAPY, AND BEHAVIORAL THERAPIES

(A) Application Exercises

1. A newly admitted client on a locked acute care mental health unit has many behavioral concerns. She refuses to attend group meetings and will not speak to other clients or attend activities on the unit. She enjoys one-to-one visits with staff, and she requests daily to take a walk out of the building with a staff member. This client's provider suggests during a treatment team meeting that behavioral therapy would be an excellent way to change this client's negative behavior, and the client agrees to try to be more cooperative. Explain how behavioral therapy could be used to help this client.

2. A client states that he is depressed and anxious because he has had to deal with role reversal with his spouse due to the permanent loss of his job. Which of the following should the nurse expect to implement for this client?

    A. Behavioral therapy

    B. Psychoanalysis

    C. Psychodynamic psychotherapy

    D. Interpersonal psychotherapy

3. A client has come to an advanced-practice nurse who practices cognitive therapy. The client's 16-year-old son has run away from home several times in the past year, and the client feels that her son's problems are her fault because she feels she is a poor mother. The nurse should use cognitive therapy to

    A. teach the client meditation to promote relaxation.

    B. help the client identify and change unrealistic thoughts.

    C. focus on the client's unconscious thoughts related to her own early childhood.

    D. give the client rewards for changing her behavior.

4. A client in an acute care mental health facility has depression and will not get out of bed. Which of the following actions should the nurse take?

    A. Give positive reinforcement for activity.

    B. Withhold rewards as long as the client remains in bed.

    C. Structure the activities of daily living to require the client's active participation.

    D. Insist that the client change his attitude and get up.

5. Match each type of therapy with the example that describes its use.

_____ Psychoanalysis

A. Staff gives a client tokens, which can be exchanged for food in a mental health facility store, when she attends group activities.

_____ Cognitive technique

B. A client discusses his dreams with the therapist.

_____ Operant conditioning

C. A client is encouraged to stop sucking his thumb by having a bitter liquid applied to it.

_____ Aversion therapy

D. A client who feels very awkward in group social situations watches a video showing some positive ways to interact in groups.

_____ Modeling

E. A client who displayed violent behavior in the past and felt negative about herself learns to think and speak about herself in more positive terms.

CHAPTER 7: PSYCHOANALYSIS, PSYCHOTHERAPY, AND BEHAVIORAL THERAPIES

 Application Exercises Answer Key

1. A newly admitted client on a locked acute care mental health unit has many behavioral concerns. She refuses to attend group meetings and will not speak to other clients or attend activities on the unit. She enjoys one-to-one visits with staff, and she requests daily to take a walk out of the building with a staff member. This client's provider suggests during a treatment team meeting that behavioral therapy would be an excellent way to change this client's negative behavior, and the client agrees to try to be more cooperative. Explain how behavioral therapy could be used to help this client.

> **Tokens or certificates given in reward for any positive change of behavior could be used to purchase items that this client likes. The client may save up a larger number of tokens or certificates for larger rewards, such as a walk outside with a staff member. Also, giving positive feedback and encouragement for positive behavior may also help.**

 NCLEX® Connection: Psychosocial Integrity, Behavioral Interventions

2. A client states that he is depressed and anxious because he has had to deal with role reversal with his spouse due to the permanent loss of his job. Which of the following therapies should the nurse expect to implement for this client?

   A. Behavioral therapy

   B. Psychoanalysis

   C. Psychodynamic psychotherapy

   D. Interpersonal psychotherapy

   Interpersonal psychotherapy will assist this client to deal with his anxiety and depression, which has resulted from the interpersonal problem of role change. A behavioral viewpoint would focus on changing the client's behavior. Psychoanalysis and psychodynamic viewpoint would focus on examining unconscious information related to the client's concern.

 NCLEX® Connection: Psychosocial Integrity, Behavioral Interventions

3. A client has come to an advanced-practice nurse who practices cognitive therapy. The client's 16-year-old son has run away from home several times in the past year, and the client feels that her son's problems are her fault because she feels she is a poor mother. The nurse should use cognitive therapy to

   A. teach the client meditation to promote relaxation.

   B. help the client identify and change unrealistic thoughts.

   C. focus on the client's unconscious thoughts related to her own early childhood.

   D. give the client rewards for changing her behavior.

   Cognitive therapy assists the client to change irrational or unrealistic thoughts to thoughts that are more realistic. Teaching a relaxation technique, or giving a reward for good behavior, are types of behavioral therapy. Focusing on unconscious thoughts related to early childhood is a technique of psychoanalysis.

 NCLEX® Connection: Psychosocial Integrity, Behavioral Interventions

4. A client in an acute care mental health facility has depression and will not get out of bed. Which of the following actions should the nurse take?

A. Give positive reinforcement for activity.

B. Withhold rewards as long as the client remains in bed.

C. Structure the activities of daily living to require the client's active participation.

D. Insist that the client change his attitude and get up.

Giving positive reinforcement is a helpful technique in gradually changing negative behaviors. The other options are negative techniques, which are unlikely to encourage any positive behavior.

Ⓝ NCLEX® Connection: Psychosocial Integrity, Behavioral Interventions

5. Match each type of therapy with the example that describes its use.

B	Psychoanalysis	A. Staff gives a client tokens, which can be exchanged for food in a mental health facility store, when she attends group activities.
E	Cognitive technique	B. A client discusses his dreams with the therapist.
A	Operant conditioning	C. A client is encouraged to stop sucking his thumb by having a bitter liquid applied to it.
C	Aversion therapy	D. A client who feels very awkward in group social situations watches a video showing some positive ways to interact in groups.
D	Modeling	E. A client who displayed violent behavior in the past and felt negative about herself learns to think and speak about herself in more positive terms.

Ⓝ NCLEX® Connection: Psychosocial Integrity, Behavioral Interventions

UNIT 2	TRADITIONAL NONPHARMACOLOGICAL THERAPIES
Chapter 8	Group and Family Therapy

Overview

- Therapy is an intensive treatment that involves open therapeutic communication with participants who are willing to be involved in therapy.

- Although individual therapy is used as an important treatment for mental illness, group and/or family therapies are also indicated as part of the treatment plan for many clients in a mental health setting.

- Group and family therapy are guided by leaders, who may employ various leadership styles:

  o Democratic – This style supports group interaction and decision making to solve problems.

  o Laissez-faire – The group process progresses without any attempt by the leader to control the direction of the group.

  o Autocratic – The leader completely controls the direction and structure of the group without allowing group interaction or decision making to solve problems.

- Examples of group therapy include stress management, chemical/alcohol dependency, medication education, understanding mental illness, and dual diagnosis groups.

Group Therapy

- Group process is the verbal and nonverbal communication that occurs within the group during group sessions.

- Group norm is the way the group behaves during sessions, and over time, it provides structure for the group. For example, a group norm could be that members raise their hand to be recognized by the leader before they speak. Another norm could be that all members sit in the same places for each session.

- Hidden agenda – Some group members (or the leader) may have goals different from the stated group goals that may disrupt group processes. For example, three members may try to embarrass another member whom they dislike.

- A subgroup is a small number of people within a larger group who function separately from the group.

- Groups may be open (new members added as old members leave) or closed (no new members added after the group is formed).

- A homogenous group is one in which all members share a certain chosen characteristic, such as diagnosis or gender. Membership of heterogeneous groups is not based on a shared chosen personal characteristic. An example of a heterogeneous group is all clients on a given unit, including a mixture of males and females with a wide range of diagnoses.

- All therapy sessions should include:

  - The use of open and clear communication

  - Cohesiveness and guidelines for the therapy session

  - Direction toward a particular goal

  - Opportunities for the development of interpersonal skills, resolution of personal and/ or family issues, and the development of appropriate, satisfying relationships

  - Encouragement of the client to maximize positive interactions, feel empowered to make decisions, and strengthen feelings of self-worth

  - Communication regarding respect among all members

  - Support, as well as education regarding things such as available community resources for support

- Group therapy goals include:

  - Sharing of common feelings and concerns

  - Sharing of stories and experiences

  - Diminishing feelings of isolation

  - Creating a community of healing and restoration

  - Providing a more cost-effective environment than that of individual therapy

- Group therapy may be used for varying age groups.

  - For children, it is in the form of play while talking about a common experience.

  - For the adolescent, it is especially valuable, as that age group typically has strong peer relationships.

  - For the older adult, group therapy helps with socialization and sharing of memories.

PHASES OF GROUP DEVELOPMENT		
PHASE	**MAJOR ISSUES**	**RESPONSIBILITIES**
Initial Phase	The purpose and goals of the group are defined.	• The group leader sets a tone of respect, trust, and confidentiality among members. • Members become acquainted with each other and with the group leader. • Termination is discussed.
Working Phase	Problem-solving skills are promoted to facilitate behavioral changes. Power and control issues may dominate in this phase.	• The group leader uses therapeutic communication to encourage group work toward meeting goals. • Members take informal roles within the group, which may interfere with, or favor, group progress toward goals.
Termination Phase	This marks the end of group sessions.	• Termination issues are discussed among group members. • The leader summarizes work of the group and individual contributions.

- Members of a group can take on any of a number of roles, including:

  o Maintenance roles – Members who take on these roles tend to help maintain the purpose and process of the group. For example, the harmonizer attempts to prevent conflict in the group.

  o Task roles – Members take on various tasks within the group process. An example of a task role is the recorder, who takes notes and/or records what occurs during each session.

  o Individual roles – These roles tend to prevent teamwork, because individuals take on roles to promote their own agenda. Examples include the dominator, who tries to control other members, and the recognition seeker, who boasts about personal achievements.

Characteristics of Families

- Families may have healthy or dysfunctional characteristics in one or more areas of functioning.

AREA OF FUNCTIONING	HEALTHY FAMILIES	DYSFUNCTIONAL FAMILIES
Communication	There are clear, understandable messages between family members, and each member is encouraged to express individual feelings and thoughts.	• One or more members use unhealthy patterns, such as: ○ Blaming – Members blame others to shift focus away from their own inadequacies. ○ Manipulating – Members use dishonesty to support their own agendas. ○ Placating – One member takes responsibility for problems in order to keep peace at all costs. ○ Distracting – A member inserts irrelevant information during attempts at problem solving.
Management	Adults of a family agree on important issues, such as rule making, finances, and plans for the future.	• Management may be chaotic, with a child making management decisions at times.
Boundaries	Boundaries are distinguishable between family roles. Clear boundaries define roles of each member and are understood by all. Each family member is able to function appropriately.	• Enmeshed boundaries – Thoughts, roles, and feelings are so blended that individual roles are unclear. • Rigid boundaries – Rules and roles are completely inflexible. These families tend to have isolated members.
Socialization	All members interact, plan, and adopt healthy ways of coping. Children learn to function as family members, as well as members of society. Members are able to change as the family grows and matures.	• Children do not learn healthy socialization skills within the family and have difficulty adapting to socialization roles of society.
Emotional/ Supportive	Emotional needs of family members are met most of the time, and members are concerned about each other. Conflict and anger do not dominate.	• Negative emotions predominate most of time. Members are isolated and afraid and do not show concern for each other.

- Other concepts related to family dysfunction include:

  o Scapegoating – A member of the family with little power is blamed for problems within the family. For example, one child who has not completed his chores may be blamed for the entire family not being able to go on an outing.

  o Triangulation – A third party is drawn into the relationship with two members whose relationship is unstable. For example, one parent may become strongly allied with a child, leaving the other parent relatively uninvolved with both.

  o Multigenerational issues – These are emotional issues or themes within a family that continue for at least three generations, such as a pattern of addiction when the family is under stress, dysfunctional grief patterns, triangulation patterns, divorce.

Family Therapy

- A family is defined as a group with reciprocal relationships in which members are committed to each other. Examples of a family vary widely and are often nontraditional, such as a family made up of a child living with her grown brother and his wife. Areas of functioning for families include management, boundaries, communication, emotional support, and socialization. Dysfunction can occur in any one or more areas.

- In family therapy, the focus is on the family as a system, rather than on each person as an individual.

- Family assessments include focused interviews and use of various family assessment tools.

- Nurses work with families to provide teaching. For example, an RN might instruct a family on medication administration, or ways to provide symptom management for a family member with a mental health disorder.

- Nurses also work to mobilize family resources, to improve communication, and to strengthen the family's ability to cope with the illness of one member.

FOCUS AND GOALS FOR INDIVIDUAL, FAMILY, AND GROUP THERAPIES		
THERAPY	FOCUS	GOALS
Individual	• Client needs and problems • The therapeutic relationship	• Make more positive individual decisions. • Make productive life decisions. • Develop a strong sense of self.
Family	• Family needs and problems within family dynamics • Improving family functioning	• Learn effective ways for dealing with mental illness within the family. • Improve understanding among family members. • Maximize positive interaction among family members.

Group	• Helping individuals develop more functional and satisfying relations within a group setting	• Goals vary depending on type of group, but clients generally:
		  ○ Discover that members share some common feelings, experiences, and thoughts.
		  ○ Experience positive behavior changes as a result of group interaction and feedback.

CHAPTER 8: GROUP AND FAMILY THERAPY

 Application Exercises

1. A client who has bipolar disorder is active in individual and family therapy. A nurse co-leads the family therapy session. The client expresses concern that his family does not understand his mental illness. The client's family expresses concern that the client may not be responding to the medication. What educational and therapeutic interventions should the nurse perform for the client and the family?

2. A nurse leading a stress management group is using a democratic leadership style. What does that mean in terms of how the group process will proceed?

3. A nurse on an acute care mental health unit is teaching members how to self-manage their psychotropic medications. Several members of the group have decided that they want the group to plan future activities for the unit and are working hard to accomplish this goal. This is an example of which of the following?

   A. Group norm

   B. Group process

   C. Subgroup

   D. Hidden agenda

4. A nurse is conducting a family therapy session. The teenage son tells the nurse that he plans ways to make his sister look bad so his parents will think of him as the better sibling, and he will therefore be allowed more priveleges. This is an example of which of the following?

   A. Placation

   B. Manipulation

   C. Blaming

   D. Distraction

CHAPTER 8: GROUP AND FAMILY THERAPY

 Application Exercises Answer Key

1. A client who has bipolar disorder is active in individual and family therapy. A nurse co-leads the family therapy session. The client expresses concern that his family does not understand his mental illness. The client's family expresses concern that the client may not be responding to the medication. What educational and therapeutic interventions should the nurse perform for the client and the family?

> **Assess further as to why the family feels the client is not responding to his medications.**
>
> **Encourage both the client and family to clarify their concerns.**
>
> **Help the client and family to find strengths on which to build.**
>
> **Maintain open communication between family members.**
>
> **Provide a safe environment for the client.**
>
> **Provide education that includes medication education.**

(N) NCLEX® Connection: Psychosocial Integrity, Support Systems

2. A nurse leading a stress management group is using a democratic leadership style. What does that mean in terms of how the group process will proceed?

> **A democratic leader supports group interaction and the decision making required to solve problems. The group should proceed with all members feeling that they have input and some control of group decisions.**

(N) NCLEX® Connection: Psychosocial Integrity, Family Dynamics

3. A nurse on an acute care mental health unit is teaching members how to self-manage their psychotropic medications. Several members of the group have decided that they want the group to plan future activities for the unit and are working hard to accomplish this goal. This is an example of which of the following?

> A. Group norm
>
> B. Group process
>
> C. Subgroup
>
> **D. Hidden agenda**
>
> A hidden agenda is when some group members have a different goal than the stated group goals; this goal is often kept hidden from the other group members. The group norm is how the group behaves during sessions and over time. Group process is the verbal and nonverbal communication that occurs within the group during group sessions. A subgroup is a small number of people within a larger group who function separately from that group.

(N) NCLEX® Connection: Psychosocial Integrity, Family Dynamics

4. A nurse is conducting a family therapy session. The teenage son tells the nurse that he plans ways to make his sister look bad so his parents will think of him as the better sibling, and he will therefore be allowed more priveleges. This is an example of which of the following?

    A. Placation

    B. Manipulation

    C. Blaming

    D. Distraction

Manipulation refers to control by dishonest influence rather than through open and honest communication. Placation is a way to keep peace in the family. Blaming is done to move the focus to another to prevent being blamed for one's own actions. Distraction is a way to prevent looking at one's own faults by introducing other issues.

(N) NCLEX® Connection: Psychosocial Integrity, Family Dynamics

UNIT 2	TRADITIONAL NONPHARMACOLOGICAL THERAPIES
Chapter 9	Stress Management

Overview

- Stress is the body's nonspecific response to any demand made upon it.

    ○ Stressors are physical or psychological factors that produce stress. Any stressor, whether it is perceived as "good" or "bad," produces a biological response in the body.

    ○ Individuals need the presence of some stressors to provide interest and purpose to life; however, too much stress or too many stressors can cause distress.

    ○ Anxiety and anger are damaging stressors that cause distress.

- General adaptation syndrome (GAS) is the body's response to an increased demand. The first stage is the initial adaptive response, also known as the "fight or flight" mechanism. If stress is prolonged, maladaptive responses can occur.

- Stress management is a person's ability to experience appropriate emotions and cope with stress.

    ○ The person who manages stress in a healthy manner is flexible and uses a variety of coping techniques or mechanisms.

    ○ Responses to stress and anxiety are affected by factors such as age, gender, culture, life experiences, and lifestyle.

    ○ The effects of stressors are cumulative. For example, the death of a family member may cause a high amount of stress. If the person experiencing that stress is also experiencing other stressful events at the same time, this could cause illness due to the cumulative effect of those stressors.

Assessment

- Protective factors increasing a person's resilience, or ability to resist the effects of stress, include:

    ○ Physical health

    ○ Strong sense of self

    ○ Religious or spiritual beliefs

    ○ Optimism

    ○ Hobbies and other outside interests

    ○ Satisfying interpersonal relationships

- ○ Strong social support systems

- ○ Humor

- Subjective and Objective Data

ACUTE STRESS (FIGHT OR FLIGHT)	PROLONGED STRESS (MALADAPTIVE RESPONSE)
Apprehension	Chronic anxiety or panic attacks
Unhappiness or sorrow	Depression, chronic pain, sleep disturbances
Decreased appetite	Weight gain or loss
Increased respiratory rate, heart rate, cardiac output, blood pressure	Increased risk for myocardial infarction, stroke
Increased metabolism and glucose use	Poor diabetes control, hypertension, fatigue, irritability, decreased ability to concentrate
Depressed immune system	Increased risk for infection

- Standardized Screening Tools

- ○ Life-changing events questionnaires, such as the Holmes and Rahe scale to measure Life Change Units, and Lazarus's Cognitive Appraisal

Collaborative Care

- Nursing Care

- ○ Most nursing care involves teaching stress-reduction strategies to clients.

- Cognitive Techniques

- ○ Cognitive reframing

- ■ The client is helped to look at irrational cognitions (thoughts) in a more realistic light and to restructure those thoughts in a more positive way.

- ■ As an example, a client may think he is "a terrible father to my daughter." A health professional, using therapeutic communication techniques, could help the person reframe that thought into a positive thought, such as, "I've made some bad mistakes as a parent, but I've learned from them and have improved my parenting skills."

- Behavioral Techniques

- ○ Relaxation techniques

- ■ Meditation includes formal meditation techniques, as well as prayer for those who believe in a higher power.

- ■ Guided imagery – The client is guided through a series of images to promote relaxation. Images vary depending on the individual. For example, one client might imagine walking on a beach, while another client might imagine himself in a position of success.

- ■ Breathing exercises are used to decrease rapid breathing and promote relaxation.

- ■ Progressive muscle relaxation (PMR) – A person trained in this method can help a client attain complete relaxation within a few minutes of time.

- ■ Physical exercise (yoga, walking, biking) causes release of endorphins that lower anxiety, promote relaxation, and have antidepressant effects.

   ○ Journal writing

- ■ Journaling has been shown to allow for a therapeutic release of stress.

- ■ This activity can help the client identify stressors and make specific plans to decrease stressors.

   ○ Priority restructuring

- ■ The client learns to prioritize differently to reduce the number of stressors impacting her.

- ■ For example, a person who is under stress due to feeling overworked might delegate some tasks to others rather than doing them all herself.

   ○ Biofeedback

- ■ A nurse or other health professional trained in this method can assist the client to gain voluntary control of such autonomic functions as heart rate and blood pressure.

   ○ Assertiveness training

- ■ The client learns to communicate in a more assertive manner in order to decrease psychological stressors.

- ■ For example, one technique teaches the client to assert his feelings by describing a situation or behavior that causes stress, stating his feelings about the behavior or situation, and then making a change. The client states, "When you keep telling me what to do, I feel angry and frustrated. I need to try making some of my own decisions."

- • Client Outcomes

   ○ The client will verbalize three stressors and ways to decrease exposure.

   ○ The client will demonstrate appropriate relaxation techniques.

   ○ The client will demonstrate assertive communication.

CHAPTER 9: STRESS MANAGEMENT

 Application Exercises

Scenario: A client, who is speaking to a nurse, describes herself as feeling "anxious and tired all the time." She cannot understand why, since she is very happy. She recently moved to the area to start a new job for a large corporation. She purchased a new and much larger home for herself and her three children, ages 5, 8, and 12. The children were all moved into new schools successfully and are making new friends. The client's family and friends are all back in the previous city where she lived, but she has been so busy with work that she has not had time to phone or write to them. The client states she has not been able to sleep and has lost weight in the 2 months since the move.

1. List the stressors that impact this client.

2. What symptoms of increased stress can be observed in this client?

3. Describe two stress-relieving activities that the nurse could recommend that would not require the client to learn new techniques, or to see a therapist or specially trained professional.

4. A client says she is experiencing increased stress because her significant other is, "pressuring me and my kids to go live with him. I love him, but I'm not ready to do that." She also states that her significant other, "keeps nagging at my oldest son, which makes me mad, since he's my son, not his." Which of the following is a coping strategy that the nurse might suggest for this client?

   A. Learn to reframe the situation.

   B. Use assertiveness techniques.

   C. Exercise regularly.

   D. Rely on the support of a close friend.

5. A client who is under a great deal of stress tells a nurse, "I just don't know how to handle all my problems. So many things are going on that I don't do anything about, because I'm not sure how to start or what to do." Based on this information, the nurse should plan for a client outcome regarding

   A. decision making.

   B. anxiety.

   C. acceptance of health status.

   D. ability to perform self-care.

CHAPTER 9: STRESS MANAGEMENT

 Application Exercises Answer Key

Scenario: A client, who is speaking to a nurse, describes herself as feeling "anxious and tired all the time." She cannot understand why, since she is very happy. She recently moved to the area to start a new job for a large corporation. She purchased a new and much larger home for herself and her three children, ages 5, 8, and 12. The children were all moved into new schools successfully and are making new friends. The client's family and friends are all back in the previous city where she lived, but she has been so busy with work that she has not had time to phone or write to them. The client states she has not been able to sleep and has lost weight in the 2 months since the move.

1. List the stressors that impact this client.

> **Recent move**
>
> **Purchase of a larger home**
>
> **Placing three children into new schools**
>
> **Sudden decrease of support systems**
>
> **New job**
>
> **Lack of free time**

 NCLEX® Connection: Psychosocial Integrity, Stress Management

2. What symptoms of increased stress can be observed in this client?

> **The client states that she feels anxious and tired all the time. She also has sleep disturbances and has had weight loss.**

 NCLEX® Connection: Psychosocial Integrity, Stress Management

3. Describe two stress-relieving activities that the nurse could recommend that would not require the client to learn new techniques, or to see a therapist or specially trained professional.

> **The client could be advised to increase physical exercise by doing things such as walking, swimming, or yoga. She could also begin to keep a journal. If she has learned meditation techniques in the past, she could try them again now.**

 NCLEX® Connection: Psychosocial Integrity, Stress Management

4. A client says she is experiencing increased stress because her significant other is, "pressuring me and my kids to go live with him. I love him, but I'm not ready to do that." She also states that her significant other, "keeps nagging at my oldest son, which makes me mad, since he's my son, not his." Which of the following is a coping strategy that the nurse might suggest for this client?

    A. Learn to reframe the situation.

    B. Use assertiveness techniques.

    C. Exercise regularly.

    D. Rely on the support of a close friend.

Assertiveness techniques would assist this client to make her feelings known and to request a change of behavior without using blaming or other negative communications. Reframing the situation is not appropriate, because the stressor does not seem to be caused by irrational thoughts. Exercise and talking to a close friend might decrease the client's stress, but they would not change the situation.

Ⓝ NCLEX® Connection: Psychosocial Integrity, Stress Management

5. A client who is under a great deal of stress tells a nurse, "I just don't know how to handle all my problems. So many things are going on that I don't do anything about, because I'm not sure how to start or what to do." Based on this information, the nurse should plan for a client outcome regarding

    A. decision making.

    B. anxiety.

    C. acceptance of health status.

    D. ability to perform self-care.

This client describes an inability to make decisions; she is experiencing negative feelings about herself and her life due to problems with decision making. The client does seem anxious, but there is no data to show that achieving self-control over anxiety would be beneficial. There is no data to prove relevance for either option C or D.

Ⓝ NCLEX® Connection: Psychosocial Integrity, Stress Management

UNIT 2   TRADITIONAL NONPHARMACOLOGICAL THERAPIES

Chapter 10   Electroconvulsive Therapy

Overview

- Electroconvulsive therapy (ECT) is an alternative somatic treatment for mental health disorders.

- ECT delivers an electrical current that produces a grand mal seizure.

- The exact mechanism of ECT is still unknown and controversial. One theory suggests that ECT may enhance the effects of neurotransmitters (serotonin, dopamine, and norepinephrine) in the brain.

Indications

- Severe Depression

  o   Clients whose symptoms are not responsive to pharmacologic treatment

  o   Clients for whom the risks of other treatments outweigh the risks of ECT, such as a client who is in her first trimester of pregnancy

  o   Clients who are actively suicidal and for whom there is a need for rapid therapeutic response

- Certain types of schizophrenia that are less responsive to neuroleptic medications, such as catatonic schizophrenia, schizoaffective disorders

- Acute Manic Episodes

  o   ECT is used for clients who have bipolar disorder with rapid cycling (four or more episodes of acute mania within 1 year) and very destructive behavior. Both of these features tend to respond poorly to lithium therapy. These clients receive ECT and then a regimen of lithium therapy.

Contraindications

- There are no absolute contraindications for this therapy if it is deemed necessary to save a client's life. However, the nurse should be aware that some clients may have medical conditions that place them at higher risk if ECT is used. These conditions include:

  o   Recent myocardial infarction

  o   History of cerebrovascular accident

  o   Cerebrovascular malformation

  o   Intracranial mass lesion

- Mental health conditions for which ECT has not been found useful include:

    o Developmental disabilities

    o Chemical dependence

    o Personality disorders

    o Situational depression

Client Outcomes

- The client is relieved of symptoms of depression.

- The client is able to perform activities of daily living.

Nursing Actions

- Preparation of the Client

    o The typical course of ECT treatment is three times a week for a total of six to 12 treatments.

    o The nurse assists with necessary teaching prior to and following informed consent, which is obtained from the client by the provider.

    o The nurse continues to provide active listening and therapeutic communication prior to the procedure and throughout the course of ECT treatments.

    o The provider discusses the procedure (including all risks and benefits, as well as a description of the procedure) with the client, and informed consent is obtained.

        □ A guardian must give consent for ECT for a client who has been declared incompetent. Some clients who have been declared incompetent require a court order.

        □ Some facilities require a separate informed consent for anesthesia, which would be obtained by an anesthesia provider.

        ■ A history and physical examination, including a neurological examination, electrocardiogram, and laboratory tests (complete blood count and other tests ordered by the provider or per facility protocol) are obtained.

    o Medication management

        ■ Any medications that affect the client's seizure threshold must be decreased or discontinued several days before the ECT procedure.

        ■ MAOIs and lithium should be discontinued 2 weeks before the ECT procedure.

    o Severe hypertension should be controlled, since a short period of hypertension occurs immediately after the ECT procedure.

    o Any cardiac conditions, such as dysrhythmias, should be monitored and treated before the procedure.

- ○ The nurse monitors the client's vital signs and mental status before and after the ECT procedure.

- ○ The nurse also assesses the client's and family's understanding and knowledge of the procedure and provides teaching as necessary.

- ○ Thirty minutes prior to the beginning of the procedure, an IM injection of atropine sulfate or robinul (Glycopyrrolate) is given to decrease secretions and counteract any vagal stimulation.

- ○ An IV line is inserted and maintained until full recovery.

- Ongoing Care

  - ▪ ECT is administered early in the morning after the client has fasted for 8 to 12 hr.

  - ▪ A bite guard should be used to prevent trauma to the oral cavity.

  - ▪ Electrodes are applied to the scalp, either unilaterally or bilaterally. The exact number and placement of electrodes is decided by the provider.

  - ▪ The client is mechanically ventilated during the procedure and receives 100% oxygen.

  - ▪ Ongoing cardiac monitoring is provided, including blood pressure, cardiac rate and rhythm, and oxygen saturation.

  - ▪ An anesthesia provider administers a short-acting anesthetic, such as methohexital (Brevital) via IV bolus.

  - ▪ A muscle relaxant, such as succinylcholine (Anectine), is then administered.

  - ▪ A cuff is placed on one leg or arm to block the muscle relaxant so that seizure activity can be monitored in the limb distal to the cuff.

  - ▪ The electrical stimulus is typically applied for 0.2 to 0.8 seconds. Seizure activity is monitored, and the duration of the seizure, which is usually 25 to 60 seconds, is documented.

  - ▪ After seizure activity has ceased, the anesthetic is discontinued.

  - ▪ The client is extubated and assisted to breathe voluntarily.

- Postprocedure Care

  - ○ When stable, the client is transferred to a recovery area where level of consciousness, cardiac status, vital signs, and oxygen saturation continue to be monitored.

  - ○ The client is positioned on his side to facilitate drainage and prevent aspiration.

  - ○ The client is usually awake and ready for transfer back to the mental health unit or other facility within 30 to 60 minutes after the procedure.

  - ○ During the recovery phase, the nurse needs to orient the client frequently, because confusion and short-term memory loss are common during this time.

  - ○ The nurse should continue to monitor the client's vital signs as indicated, and mental status for memory loss.

Complications

- Memory Loss and Confusion

    o Short-term memory loss, confusion, and disorientation may occur immediately following the procedure. Memory loss may persist for several weeks. Whether or not ECT causes permanent memory loss is controversial.

    o Nursing actions

        ▪ Provide frequent orientation.

        ▪ Provide a safe environment to prevent injury.

        ▪ Assist the client with personal hygiene as needed.

    o Client education

        ▪ Explain to the client and family that memory loss is typically short term.

        ▪ Assist the client with memory during this period.

            ▫ Place a clock in the client's room.

            ▫ Label the client's room location.

- Reactions to Anesthesia

    o Nursing Actions

        ▪ Provide continuous monitoring during the procedure and in the immediate postrecovery phase.

- ECG Changes

    o The client's baseline heart rate is expected to increase by 25% during the procedure and early recovery.

    o Blood pressure may initially fall and then rise during the procedure. The elevated blood pressure should resolve shortly after the procedure.

    o Nursing actions

        ▪ Monitor the client's vital signs regularly per protocol.

        ▪ Orient the client as necessary.

- Headache, muscle soreness, and nausea can occur during and following the immediate recovery period

    o Nursing actions

        ▪ Observe the client to determine the degree of discomfort.

        ▪ Administer antiemetic and analgesic medications as needed.

    o Client education

        ▪ Explain the reason for the symptoms to the client.

        ▪ Encourage the client to contact the nurse regarding these symptoms.

CHAPTER 10: ELECTROCONVULSIVE THERAPY

(A) Application Exercises

Scenario: A client who has major depression and has not responded to antidepressant medications is admitted to an acute care mental health facility for ECT. The client is voluntarily receiving ECT; however, he and his family have concerns regarding the treatment.

1. List care to be provided by the nurse for the client and his family.

2. The client's mother says, "We hear that people are really confused after ECT. Why should he have this treatment if he'll act like he has Alzheimer's afterward?" How should the nurse respond?

3. For which of the following should a nurse monitor during or immediately following an ECT procedure? (Select all that apply.)

_____ Hypotension

_____ Heart rate changes

_____ Intestinal obstruction

_____ Confusion

_____ Nausea

_____ Hypertension

4. Which of the following is a possible indication for ECT?

A. Borderline personality disorder

B. Suicidal ideation caused by the recent loss of a significant other

C. Bipolar disorder with mania that has occurred six times in the past year

D. Paranoid schizophrenia and a moderate developmental disability

CHAPTER 10: ELECTROCONVULSIVE THERAPY

 Application Exercises Answer Key

Scenario: A client who has major depression and has not responded to antidepressant medications is admitted to an acute care mental health facility for ECT. The client is voluntarily receiving ECT; however, he and his family have concerns regarding the treatment.

1. List care to be provided by the nurse for the client and his family.

> Assess the client's medical history.
>
> Collaborate with the provider regarding specific teaching for the ECT procedure as it applies to the client.
>
> Explain adverse reactions of the procedure to the client and family in short, easy-to-understand explanations.
>
> Be consistent when explaining procedures.
>
> Educate the client and family on safety precautions and maintenance of self-care needs. Listen to the concerns and fears of the client and his family.
>
> Help the client and the family to make and adhere to schedules for future ECT appointments.

> **NCLEX® Connection:** Reduction of Risk Potential, Potential for Complications of Diagnostic Tests/Treatments/Procedures

2. The client's mother says, "We hear that people are really confused after ECT. Why should he have this treatment if he'll act like he has Alzheimer's afterward?" How should the nurse respond?

> A client who undergoes ECT is usually confused only for a short time immediately following the procedure. There may be some longer-term memory loss for a few weeks afterward, but it is not at all like that associated with Alzheimer's disease. The health care team members will be reorienting the client, both in the recovery room and on the unit, and the provider will be informed of any mental status effects of the procedure.

> **NCLEX® Connection:** Reduction of Risk Potential, Potential for Complications of Diagnostic Tests/Treatments/Procedures

3. For which of the following should a nurse monitor during or immediately following an ECT procedure? (Select all that apply.)

___X___ **Hypotension**

___X___ **Heart rate changes**

_____ Intestinal obstruction

___X___ **Confusion**

___X___ **Nausea**

___X___ **Hypertension**

All of the above may potentially occur during or following ECT, with the exception of intestinal obstruction, which should not occur with this procedure.

 NCLEX® Connection: Reduction of Risk Potential, Potential for Complications of Diagnostic Tests/Treatments/Procedures

4. Which of the following is a possible indication for ECT?

A. Borderline personality disorder

B. Suicidal ideation caused by the recent loss of a significant other

C. Bipolar disorder with mania that has occurred six times in the past year

D. Paranoid schizophrenia and a moderate developmental disability

A client who has bipolar disorder, rapid cycling, and destructive mania is a possible candidate for ECT. Clients who are not typically good candidates for ECT include those with personality disorders, situational depression, chemical dependency, or a developmental disability.

 NCLEX® Connection: Reduction of Risk Potential, Potential for Complications of Diagnostic Tests/Treatments/Procedures

UNIT 3: PSYCHOBIOLOGIC DISORDERS

- Anxiety Disorders
- Depression
- Bipolar Disorders
- Schizophrenia
- Personality Disorders
- Cognitive Disorders
- Chemical and Other Dependencies
- Eating Disorders

NCLEX® CONNECTIONS

When reviewing the chapters in this unit, keep in mind the relevant sections of the NCLEX® outline, in particular:

CLIENT NEEDS: PSYCHOSOCIAL INTEGRITY

Relevant topics/tasks include:
- Crisis Intervention
  - Identify the client in crisis.
- Behavioral Interventions
  - Assist the client to develop and use strategies to decrease anxiety.
- Mental Health Concepts
  - Recognize signs and symptoms of acute and chronic mental illness.
  - Assess the client for alterations in mood, judgment, cognition, and reasoning.
- Therapeutic Communication
  - Encourage the client to verbalize feelings.
- Therapeutic Environment
  - Provide a therapeutic environment for clients with emotional/behavioral issues.

CLIENT NEEDS: PHARMACOLOGICAL AND PARENTERAL THERAPIES

Relevant topics/tasks include:
- Adverse Effects/Contraindications/Side Effects/Interactions
  - Assess the client for actual or potential side effects and adverse effects of medications.
- Expected Actions/Outcomes
  - Obtain information about prescribed medication for the client.

UNIT 3	PSYCHOBIOLOGIC DISORDERS
Chapter 11	Anxiety Disorders

Overview

- Anxiety is a response to stress. Higher levels of anxiety result in behavior changes. Anxiety tends to be persistent and is often disabling.

- Anxiety levels can be mild (restlessness, increased motivation, irritability), moderate (agitation, muscle tightness), severe (inability to function, ritualistic behavior, unresponsive), or panic (distorted perception, loss of rational thought, immobility).

- The various anxiety disorders recognized and defined by the DSM-IV-TR include:

    o Panic disorder – The client experiences recurrent panic attacks.

    o Phobias – The client fears a specific object or situation to an unreasonable level.

    o Obsessive compulsive disorder (OCD) – The client has intrusive thoughts of unrealistic obsessions and tries to control these thoughts with compulsive behaviors (for example, repetitive cleaning of a particular object or washing of hands).

    o Generalized anxiety disorder (GAD) – The client exhibits uncontrollable, excessive worry for more than 6 months.

    o Stress-related disorders include:

        ■ Acute stress disorder – Exposure to a traumatic event causes numbing, detachment, and amnesia about the event for not more than 4 weeks following the event.

        ■ Posttraumatic stress disorder (PTSD) – Exposure to a traumatic event causes intense fear, horror, flashbacks, feelings of detachment and foreboding, restricted affect, and impairment for longer than 1 month after the event. Symptoms may last for years.

- Defense mechanisms are cognitive distortions used to deal with stress, and their use is common in individuals with anxiety disorders. Commonly used defense mechanisms include displacement, undoing, reaction formation, intellectualization, isolation, and repression.

Assessment

- Risk Factors

    o Except for OCD, which has equal prevalence in men and women, anxiety disorders are much more likely to occur in women.

    o Exposure to a traumatic event or experience, such as military combat or threat of death of a loved one, can precipitate an anxiety disorder.

- o Anxiety can be due to an acute medical condition, such as pulmonary embolism. It is important that symptoms of anxiety be assessed in the appropriate medical facility to rule out a physical cause.

  - o Substance-induced anxiety can be related to current use of a chemical substance, or to withdrawal symptoms from a substance, such as alcohol.

- Subjective and Objective Data

  - o Panic disorder

    - Episodes typically last 15 to 30 min.

    - Four or more of the following symptoms are present:

      - □ Palpitations

      - □ Shortness of breath

      - □ Choking or smothering sensation

      - □ Chest pain

      - □ Nausea

      - □ Feelings of depersonalization

      - □ Fear of dying or insanity

      - □ Chills or hot flashes

    - The client may experience behavior changes and/or persistent worries about when the next attack will occur.

    - The client may begin to experience agoraphobia due to a fear of being in places where previous panic attacks occurred. For example, if previous attacks occurred while driving, the client may stop driving. If attacks continue while walking or taking alternative transportation, the client may remain at home.

  - o Phobias

    - Social phobia – The client has a fear of embarrassment, is unable to perform in front of others, has a dread of social situations, believes that others are judging him negatively, and has impaired relationships.

    - Agoraphobia – The client avoids being outside and has an impaired ability to work or perform duties.

    - Specific phobias

      - □ The client has a fear of specific objects, such as spiders, snakes, strangers.

      - □ The client has a fear of specific experiences, such as flying, being in the dark, riding in an elevator, being in an enclosed space.

○ Obsessive compulsive disorder (OCD) – The client has intrusive thoughts of unrealistic obsessions and tries to control these thoughts with compulsive behaviors, such as repetitive cleaning of a particular object or washing of hands.

■ Clients who engage in constant ritualistic behaviors may have difficulty meeting self-care needs, such as personal hygiene, grooming, nutrition, fluid intake, elimination, sleep.

■ If rituals include constant handwashing or cleaning, skin damage and infection may occur.

○ Generalized anxiety disorder (GAD) – The client exhibits uncontrollable, excessive worry for more than 6 months.

■ GAD causes significant impairment in one or more areas of functioning, such as work-related duties.

■ At least three of the following physical symptoms are present:

□ Fatigue

□ Restlessness

□ Problems with concentration

□ Irritability

□ Increased muscle tension

□ Sleep disturbances

○ Stress-related disorders

	ACUTE STRESS DISORDER	PTSD
Precipitating event	• In both disorders, the client witnesses or experiences an actual event that threatens severe injury or death to the client or others. • The client responds with fear, helplessness, or horror to the event.	
First symptoms	Symptoms occur within 4 weeks of the traumatic event.	The onset of symptoms is delayed at least 3 months from the precipitating event, and onset may not occur until years afterward.
Duration	Symptoms last from 2 days to 4 weeks.	Symptoms last more than 1 month. • Acute PTSD – duration less than 3 months • Chronic PTSD – duration more than 3 months

	ACUTE STRESS DISORDER	PTSD
Re-experience of the event	The client persistently re-experiences the event through: • Distress when reminded of the event • Dreams or images • Reliving through flashbacks	The client persistently re-experiences the event through: • Recurrent, intrusive recollection of the event • Dreams or images • Reliving through flashbacks, illusions, or hallucinations
Symptoms	• Dissociative symptoms, such as amnesia of the trauma event, absent emotional response, decreased awareness of surroundings, depersonalization • Symptoms of severe anxiety, such as irritability, sleep disturbance	• Symptoms of increased arousal, such as irritability, difficulty with concentration, sleep disturbance • Avoidance of stimuli associated with trauma, such as avoiding people, inability to show feelings

- Standardized Screening Tools

    o Hamilton Rating Scale for Anxiety

    o Modified Speilberger State Anxiety Scale

Collaborative Care

- Nursing Care

    o Provide a structured interview to keep the client focused on the present.

    o Provide safety and comfort to the client during the crisis period of these disorders, as clients in severe- to panic-level anxiety are unable to problem solve and focus.

    o Remain with the client during the worst of the anxiety to provide reassurance.

    o Provide a safe environment for other clients and staff.

    o Provide milieu therapy that employs the following:

        ■ A structured environment for physical safety and predictability

        ■ Monitoring for, and protection from, self-harm

        ■ Daily activities that encourage the client to share and be cooperative

        ■ Use of therapeutic communication skills, such as open-ended questions, to help the client express feelings of anxiety, and to validate and acknowledge those feelings

        ■ Client participation in decision making regarding care

- ○ Use relaxation techniques with the client as needed for symptoms of pain, muscle tension, and feelings of anxiety.

- ○ Instill hope for positive outcomes (but avoid false reassurance).

- ○ Enhance client self-esteem by encouraging positive statements and discussing past achievements.

- ○ Assist the client to identify defense mechanisms that interfere with recovery.

- ○ Postpone health teaching until after acute anxiety subsides. Clients experiencing a panic attack or severe anxiety are unable to concentrate or learn.

- ○ Specific therapies include:

    - ■ Cognitive reframing – The anxiety response can be decreased by changing cognitive distortions. This therapy assists the client to identify negative thoughts that produce anxiety, examine the cause, and develop supportive ideas that replace negative self-talk.

    - ■ Behavioral therapies teach clients ways to decrease anxiety or avoidant behavior and allow an opportunity to practice techniques.

        - □ Relaxation training can be used to control pain, tension, and anxiety.

        - □ Modeling allows a client to see a demonstration of appropriate behavior in a stressful situation. The goal of therapy is that the client will be able to imitate the behavior.

        - □ Systematic desensitization begins with mastering of relaxation techniques. Then, a client is exposed to increasing levels of an anxiety-producing stimulus (either imagined or real) and uses relaxation to overcome the resulting anxiety. The goal of therapy is that the client will be able to tolerate a greater and greater level of the stimulus until anxiety no longer interferes with functioning.

        - □ Flooding involves exposing the client to a great deal of an undesirable stimulus in an attempt to turn off the anxiety response.

        - □ Response prevention focuses on preventing the client from performing a compulsive behavior with the intent that anxiety will diminished.

        - □ Thought stopping teaches a client to say "stop" when negative thoughts or compulsive behaviors arise, and substitute a positive thought. The goal of therapy is that with time, the client uses the command silently.

    - ■ Group and family therapy, for clients with PTSD.

- • Medications

    - ○ Antidepressants, such as sertraline (Zoloft), amitriptyline (Elavil); sedative hypnotic anxiolytics, such as diazepam (Valium); serotonin norepinephrine reuptake inhibitors, such as venlafaxine (Effexor); and nonbarbiturate anxiolytics, such as buspirone (BuSpar); are used to manage anxiety.

    - ○ Other medications that can be used to treat anxiety disorders include beta blockers and antihistamines to decrease anxiety. Anticonvulsants are used as mood stabilizers for the client who is experiencing anxiety.

- Care After Discharge
  - Client education
    - Educate the client regarding identification of signs and symptoms of anxiety.
    - Instruct the client to notify the provider of worsening symptoms and to not adjust medication dosages. Warn the client against stopping or increasing medication without consultation with the provider.
    - Assist the client to evaluate coping mechanisms that work and do not work for controlling the anxiety, and assist the client to learn new methods. Use of alternative stress relief and coping mechanisms may increase medication effectiveness and decrease the need for medication in most cases.

Client Outcomes

- The client will verbalize decreased feelings of anxiety.
- The client will be rested upon awakening.
- The client will develop realistic goals for the future.
- The client will regularly attend a support group.
- The client will demonstrate appropriate use of relaxation techniques.

CHAPTER 11: ANXIETY DISORDERS

 Application Exercises

1. When assessing a client who states that she has been dealing with constant anxiety for the past few weeks, the nurse should use which of the following communication techniques?

    A. Ask open-ended questions.

    B. Provide reassurance.

    C. Minimize the client's symptoms.

    D. Offer advice.

2. During an assessment, a client tells the nurse, "I remove my old makeup and apply new makeup every hour or so because I look horrible." The nurse should understand that this behavior is consistent with which of the following disorders?

    A. Generalized anxiety disorder

    B. Panic disorder

    C. Obsessive compulsive disorder

    D. Posttraumatic stress disorder

3. Which of the following is an appropriate nursing intervention for a client experiencing a panic attack?

    A. Teach the client relaxation techniques.

    B. Show the client how to change his behavior.

    C. Distract the client with a television show.

    D. Stay with the client and remain quiet.

4. A nurse observes a client who is pacing and wringing his hands. The client states being worried since last year that his son will die a horrible death. The nurse should understand that these symptoms are consistent with which of the following disorders?

    A. Generalized anxiety disorder

    B. A specific phobia

    C. Posttraumatic stress disorder

    D. Obsessive compulsive disorder

5. A client hospitalized in an acute care mental health facility ritualistically cleans the sink in her bathroom multiple times daily. The outcome identified by the treatment team is that the client should use more effective coping measures. To achieve the desired outcome, the nurse should

    A. suggest that the client work with the maintenance staff in cleaning unit bathrooms.

    B. focus on the client's symptoms rather than on her feelings.

    C. encourage the client to participate in a variety of unit activities.

    D. enforce a strict schedule for the client's use of the bathroom.

6. Match the specific anxiety disorder with its characteristics.

_____ Obsessive compulsive disorder

_____ Panic disorder

_____ Generalized anxiety disorder

_____ Agoraphobia

_____ Social phobia

_____ Posttraumatic stress disorder

A. Traumatic event causing symptoms months after the event takes place

B. Excessive worries for more than 6 months

C. Fear of speaking or interacting in public

D. Symptoms including chest pain, palpitations, a feeling that one is about to die

E. Fear of being out in open spaces

F. Ritualistic compulsions and recurrent thoughts

CHAPTER 11: ANXIETY DISORDERS

 Application Exercises Answer Key

1. When assessing a client who states that she has been dealing with constant anxiety for the past few weeks, the nurse should use which of the following communication techniques?

    A. Ask open-ended questions.

    B. Provide reassurance.

    C. Minimize the client's symptoms.

    D. Offer advice.

    Open-ended questions allow the client to tell the nurse about her anxiety. Providing reassurance, minimizing the symptoms, and offering advice are examples of nontherapeutic communication that may be dismissive of the client's concerns.

 NCLEX® Connection: Psychosocial Integrity, Therapeutic Communications

2. During an assessment, a client tells the nurse, "I remove my old makeup and apply new makeup every hour or so because I look horrible." The nurse should understand that this behavior is consistent with which of the following disorders?

    A. Generalized anxiety disorder

    B. Panic disorder

    C. Obsessive compulsive disorder

    D. Posttraumatic stress disorder

    Obsessive compulsive disorder is characterized by repetitive, unreasonable behaviors used to reduce anxiety, such as the hourly reapplication of makeup. Generalized anxiety disorder is characterized by excessive worry over multiple concerns for more than 6 months. In panic disorder, the client has recurrent panic attacks. Posttraumatic stress disorder causes repeated re-experiencing of a traumatic event.

 NCLEX® Connection: Psychosocial Integrity, Mental Health Concepts

3. Which of the following is an appropriate nursing intervention for a client experiencing a panic attack?

    A. Teach the client relaxation techniques.

    B. Show the client how to change his behavior.

    C. Distract the client with a television show.

    D. Stay with the client and remain quiet.

    During a panic attack, the client is unable to think about anything except the symptoms being experienced. The nurse should stay with the client. The client will not be able to be distracted and will not be able to concentrate in order to learn new material. Other interventions should be postponed until after the attack.

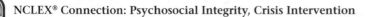 NCLEX® Connection: Psychosocial Integrity, Crisis Intervention

RN MENTAL HEALTH NURSING

4. A nurse observes a client who is pacing and wringing his hands. The client states being worried since last year that his son will die a horrible death. The nurse should understand that these symptoms are consistent with which of the following disorders?

    A. Generalized anxiety disorder

    B. A specific phobia

    C. Posttraumatic stress disorder

    D. Obsessive-compulsive disorder

Generalized anxiety disorder is characterized by worry of long duration and without cause. The symptoms described are not those of a specific phobia. Posttraumatic stress disorder causes repeated re-experiencing of a traumatic event. Obsessive compulsive disorder is characterized by repetitive unreasonable behaviors, such as handwashing, to reduce anxiety.

 NCLEX® Connection: Psychosocial Integrity, Mental Health Concepts

5. A client hospitalized in an acute care mental health facility ritualistically cleans the sink in her bathroom multiple times daily. The outcome identified by the treatment team is that the client should use more effective coping measures. To achieve the desired outcome, the nurse should

    A. suggest that the client work with the maintenance staff in cleaning unit bathrooms.

    B. focus on the client's symptoms rather than on the client's feelings.

    C. encourage the client to participate in a variety of unit activities.

    D. enforce a strict schedule for the client's use of the bathroom.

Encouraging the client to participate in unit activities and become involved with other people helps to decrease involvement in the ritualistic behavior and encourages coping skills. Encouraging the client to clean focuses on the ritual. The nurse should focus on client feelings rather than on symptoms, because these feelings are what cause the symptoms. Enforcing a strict schedule for the client's use of the bathroom is punitive and will not assist her to use more effective coping measures.

 NCLEX® Connection: Psychosocial Integrity, Therapeutic Environment

6. Match the specific anxiety disorder with its characteristics.

F	Obsessive compulsive disorder	A. Traumatic event causing symptoms months after the event takes place
D	Panic disorder	B. Excessive worries for more than 6 months
B	Generalized anxiety disorder	C. Fear of speaking or interacting in public
E	Agoraphobia	D. Symptoms including chest pain, palpitations, a feeling that one is about to die
C	Social phobia	E. Fear of being out in open spaces
A	Posttraumatic stress disorder	F. Ritualistic compulsions and recurrent thoughts

 NCLEX® Connection: Psychosocial Integrity, Mental Health Concepts

UNIT 3	PSYCHOBIOLOGIC DISORDERS
Chapter 12	Depression

Overview

- Depression is a mood (affective) disorder that is a widespread issue, ranking high among causes of disability.

- Depression may be comorbid with the following:

  o Anxiety disorders

    ▪ These disorders are comorbid with 70% of major depressive disorders, the combination of which makes a client's prognosis poorer, with a higher risk for suicide and disability.

  o Schizophrenia

  o Substance abuse

    ▪ Clients often abuse substances in order to relieve symptoms and/or self-treat mental health disorders.

  o Eating disorders

  o Personality disorders

- A client with depression may be at risk for suicide, especially if he has a family or personal history of suicide attempts, comorbid anxiety disorder or panic attacks, comorbid substance abuse or psychosis, poor self-esteem, a lack of social support, or a chronic medical condition.

- Depressive disorders recognized and defined by the DSM-IV-TR include:

  o Major depressive disorder (MDD) is a single episode or recurrent episodes of unipolar depression (not associated with mood swings from major depression to mania) resulting in a significant change in a client's normal functioning (social, occupational, self-care) accompanied by at least five of the following specific symptoms, which must occur almost every day for a minimum of 2 weeks, and last most of the day:

    ▪ Depressed mood

    ▪ Difficulty sleeping or excessive sleeping

    ▪ Indecisiveness

    ▪ Decreased ability to concentrate

    ▪ Suicidal ideation

- Increase or decrease in motor activity
- Inability to feel pleasure
- Increase or decrease in weight of more than 5% of total body weight over 1 month

  ○ MDD may be further diagnosed in the DSM-IV-TR with a more specific classification (specifier), including:

  - Psychotic features – the presence of auditory hallucinations (for example, voices telling the client she is sinful) or the presence of delusions (for example, client thinking that she has a fatal disease)
  - Atypical features – changes in appetite or weight gain, excessive daytime sleepiness
  - Postpartum onset – a depressive episode that begins within 4 weeks of childbirth (known as postpartum depression) and may include delusions, which may put the newborn infant at high risk of being harmed by the mother
  - Seasonal characteristics – seasonal affective disorder (SAD), which occurs during winter and may be treated with light therapy
  - Chronic features – a depressive episode that lasts over 2 years

  ○ Dysthymic disorder is a milder form of depression that usually has an early onset, such as in childhood or adolescence, and lasts at least 2 years in length for adults (1 year in length for children). Dysthymic disorder contains at least three symptoms of depression and may, later in life, become major depressive disorder.

  ○ Care of a client with MDD will mirror the phase of the disease that the client is experiencing:

PHASE	CHARACTERISTICS	TREATMENT
Acute	Severe symptoms of depression	• Treatment is generally 6 to 12 weeks in duration. • Hospitalization may be required. • Reduction of depressive symptoms is the goal of treatment. • Suicide potential is determined and safety precautions implemented. • One-to-one observation may be indicated.
Maintenance	Increased ability to function	• Treatment is generally 4 to 9 months in duration. • Relapse prevention through education, medication therapy, and psychotherapy is the goal of treatment.
Continuation	Remission of symptoms	• This phase may last for years. • Prevention of future depressive episodes is the goal of treatment.

Assessment

- Risk Factors

    o Family history and a previous personal history of depression are the most significant risk factors.

    o Depressive disorders are twice as common in females between the ages of 15 and 40 than in males.

    o Depression is very common among clients over age 65, but the disorder is more difficult to recognize in the older adult client and may go untreated. It is important to differentiate between early dementia and depression. Some symptoms of depression that may look like dementia are memory loss, confusion, and behavioral problems, such as social isolation or agitation. Clients may seek health care for somatic symptoms that are manifestations of untreated depression.

    o A neurotransmitter deficiency, such as a serotonin deficiency, that affects mood, sexual behavior, sleep cycles, hunger, and pain perception can be a risk factor for depression.

    o Other risk factors include:

        ▪ Stressful life events

        ▪ Presence of a medical illness

        ▪ Being a female in the postpartum period

        ▪ Poor social support network

        ▪ Comorbid substance abuse

    o Depression occurs throughout all groups of people. There are no specific risk factors for ethnicity, education, income, or marital status.

    o Depression may be the primary disorder, or it may be a response to another physical or mental health disorder.

- Subjective Data

    o Anergia (lack of energy)

    o Anhedonia (lack of pleasure in normal activities)

    o Anxiety

    o Reports of sluggishness (most common), or feeling unable to relax and sit still

    o Vegetative signs, which include a change in eating patterns (usually anorexia in MDD, and increased intake in dysthymia), change in bowel habits (usually constipation), sleep disturbances, and decreased interest in sexual activity

    o Somatic reports, such as fatigue, gastrointestinal symptoms, pain

- Objective Data

    o Physical assessment findings

        ▪ Affect – The client most often looks sad with blunted affect.

        ▪ The client exhibits poor grooming and lack of hygiene.

- Psychomotor retardation (slowed physical movement, slumped posture) is more common, but psychomotor agitation (restlessness, pacing, finger tapping) can also occur.

- The client becomes socially isolated, showing little or no effort to interact.

- Slowed speech, decreased verbalization, delayed response – The client may seem too tired even to speak.

- Standardized Screening Tools

  - Hamilton Depression Scale

  - Beck Depression Inventory

  - Geriatric Depression Scale (short form)

  - Zung's Self-Rating Depression Scale

  - A confidential screening tool can be found at http://www.depression-screening.org.

Collaborative Care

- Nursing Care

  - Milieu Therapy

    - Self-care – Monitor the client's ability to perform activities of daily living and encourage independence as much as possible.

    - Communication

      - Relate therapeutically to the client who is unable or unwilling to communicate.

        ‣ Make time to be with the client, even if he does not speak.

        ‣ Make observations rather than asking direct questions, which may cause anxiety in the client. For example, the nurse might say, "I noticed that you attended the unit group meeting today," rather than asking, "Did you enjoy the group meeting?"Give directions in simple, concrete sentences, since the client with depression may have difficulty focusing on and comprehending long sentences.

        ‣ Give the client sufficient time to respond when holding a conversation; the client's response time may be greatly slowed.

    - Maintenance of a safe environment

    - Counseling – This may include individual counseling to assist with the following:

      - Problem solving

      - Increasing coping abilities

      - Changing negative thinking to positive

      - Increasing self-esteem

      - Assertiveness training

      - Using available community resources

- Medications

    - Antidepressants

        - Client teaching for all antidepressants

            - Do not discontinue medication suddenly.

            - Medications may take 1 to 3 weeks for therapeutic effects for initial response with up to 2 months for maximal response.

            - Avoid hazardous activities, such as driving or operating heavy equipment/machinery.

MEDICATION CLASSIFICATION/EXAMPLE	CLIENT TEACHING
Selective Serotonin Reuptake Inhibitors (SSRIs) • Citalopram (Celexa) • Fluoxetine (Prozac) • Sertraline (Zoloft)	• Side effects may include nausea, headache, and CNS stimulation (agitation, insomnia, anxiety). • Sexual dysfunction may occur. Notify primary care provider if effects are intolerable. • Follow healthy diet, as weight gain can occur with long-term use.
Tricyclic Antidepressants • Amitriptyline (Elavil)	• Advise client to change positions slowly to minimize dizziness from orthostatic hypotension.
Monoamine Oxidase Inhibitors (MAOIs) • Phenelzine (Nardil)	• To minimize anticholinergic effects, advise the client to chew sugarless gum, eat foods high in fiber, and increase fluid intake to 2 to 3 L/day from food and beverage sources. • Advise the client to avoid foods with tyramine (ripe avocados or figs, fermented or smoked meats, liver, dried or cured fish, most cheeses, some beer and wine, and protein dietary supplements).
Sedative Hypnotic Anxiolytics (Benzodiazepines) • Diazepam (Valium) • Lorazepam (Ativan)	• Watch for CNS depression, such as sedation, lightheadedness, ataxia, and decreased cognitive function. • Avoid the use of other CNS depressants, such as alcohol. • Avoid hazardous activities (driving, operating heavy equipment/machinery). • Caffeine interferes with the desired effects of the medication. • Advise the client who has been taking these medications regularly and in high doses to taper the dose over several weeks to prevent withdrawal symptoms.
Serotonin Norepinephrine Reuptake Inhibitors • Venlafaxine (Effexor)	• Side effects include nausea, weight gain, and sexual dysfunction.
Nonbarbiturate Anxiolytics • Buspirone (BuSpar)	• Onset of therapeutic effects may take 2 to 4 weeks. • Nonbarbiturate anxiolytics may be used for long-term management of depression. • This class of medication does not cause CNS depression.

- Interdisciplinary Care

  o Psychotherapy by a trained therapist may include individual cognitive-behavioral therapy, group therapy, and family therapy.

- Alternative or Complementary Therapies

  o St. John's Wort – a plant product (*Hypericum perforatum*), not regulated by the United States FDA, is taken by some individuals to relieve symptoms of mild depression.

    ▪ Nursing considerations

      □ Adverse effects include photosensitivity, skin rash, rapid heart rate, gastrointestinal distress, and abdominal pain.

      □ St. John's Wort can increase or reduce levels of some medications if taken concurrently. The client should inform the provider if taking St. John's Wort.

      □ Medication interactions – Potentially fatal serotonin syndrome can result if St. John's Wort is taken with SSRIs; MAOIs; atypical antidepressants, such as nefazodone (Serzone) or venlafaxine (Effexor); and tricyclic antidepressants, such as amitriptyline (Elavil) and clomipramine (Anafranil). Foods containing tyramine should be avoided.

  o Light therapy – First-line treatment for seasonal affective disorder (SAD), light therapy inhibits nocturnal secretion of melatonin.

    ▪ Exposure of the face to 10,000-lux light box 30 minutes a day, once or in 2 divided doses

- Therapeutic Procedures

  o Electroconvulsive therapy (ECT) can be useful for some clients with depression.

    ▪ Nursing Actions

      □ A specially trained nurse is responsible for monitoring the client before and after this therapy.

  o Transcranial magnetic stimulation (TMS) is a new therapy using electromagnetic stimulation of the brain; it may be helpful for depression that is resistant to other forms of treatment.

  o Vagus nerve stimulation (VNS therapy system) is an implanted device that stimulates the vagus nerve. It can be used for clients who have depression that is resistant to at least four antidepressant medications.

- Care After Discharge
  - Continuation phase followed by maintenance phase
    - Client education
      - Review signs and symptoms of depression with client and family members in order to identify relapse.
      - Reinforce intended effects and potential side effects of medication.
      - Explain the benefits of the client's adherence to therapy.
      - Exercise – Thirty minutes of exercise daily for 3 to 5 days each week improves symptoms of depression and may help to prevent relapse. Even shorter intervals of exercise are helpful. Exercise should be regarded as an adjunct to other therapies for the client with major depressive disorder.

CHAPTER 12: DEPRESSION

 Application Exercises

Scenario: A 35-year-old female client is newly admitted to an acute care mental health facility for her third episode of major depressive disorder. She is a school teacher who is currently on medical leave. She lives at home with her husband and two school-age children, but she has stopped cooking, doing housework, and grooming herself or the children during the past 3 weeks. She says she has a complete lack of energy to do anything, a lack of appetite with a 5-lb weight loss, constipation, abdominal pain, and an inability to sleep more than 5 hr each night (wakes up early and cannot get back to sleep). During the admission interview, she says to the nurse, "It would be better for my family if I just wasn't around ever again. I'm no good for them anymore, and I have no control over any of my life."

1. Which of the following are risk factors for depression for this client? (Select all that apply.)

    _____ Age

    _____ Having two school-age children

    _____ Prior history of depressive episodes

    _____ Being married

2. The client's husband tells the nurse, "I hope my wife will be able to take her St. John's Wort here in the hospital." Which of the client's symptoms could be related to taking St. John's Wort?

3. The client has recently begun taking the SSRI paroxetine (Paxil). What should the nurse teach the client and spouse about taking this medication concurrently with St. John's Wort?

4. Which of the following interventions is the highest priority regarding management of this client's care?

    A. Placing the client on one-to-one observation

    B. Assisting the client to perform morning care

    C. Encouraging the client to participate in unit activities

    D. Teaching the client about medication side effects

5. A nurse is interviewing a 25-year-old client diagnosed with dysthymia. Which of the following findings should the nurse expect?

    A. There are wide fluctuations in mood.

    B. There is no evidence of suicidal ideation.

    C. The symptoms last for at least 2 years.

    D. There is an inflated sense of self-esteem.

CHAPTER 12: DEPRESSION

 Application Exercises Answer Key

Scenario: A 35-year-old female client is newly admitted to an acute care mental health facility for her third episode of major depressive disorder. She is a school teacher who is currently on medical leave. She lives at home with her husband and two school-age children, but she has stopped cooking, doing housework, and grooming herself or the children during the past 3 weeks. She says she has a complete lack of energy to do anything, a lack of appetite with a 5-lb weight loss, constipation, abdominal pain, and an inability to sleep more than 5 hr each night (wakes up early and cannot get back to sleep). During the admission interview, she says to the nurse, "It would be better for my family if I just wasn't around ever again. I'm no good for them anymore, and I have no control over any of my life."

1. Which of the following are risk factors for depression for this client? (Select all that apply.)

   X   **Age**

          Having two school-age children

   X   **Prior history of depressive episodes**

          Being married

    Depression is most common in females between the ages of 15 and 40. A prior depressive episode places this client at risk for another episode. Having two small children, being a school teacher, and being married are not risk factors for depression.

 NCLEX® Connection: Psychosocial Integrity, Crisis Intervention

2. The client's husband tells the nurse, "I hope my wife will be able to take her St. John's Wort here in the hospital." Which of the client's symptoms could be related to taking St. John's Wort?

    Abdominal pain is one adverse reaction associated with the use of St. John's Wort. Others possible reactions include photosensitivity, skin rash, rapid heart rate, and gastrointestinal upset.

 NCLEX® Connection: Pharmacological and Parenteral Therapies, Adverse Effects/ Contraindications/Side Effects/Interactions

3. The client has recently begun taking the SSRI paroxetine (Paxil). What should the nurse teach the client and spouse about taking this medication concurrently with St. John's Wort?

    Combining any SSRI antidepressant with St. John's Wort can cause serotonin syndrome, a serious condition that includes high fever, hypertension, and delirium. The client should not continue to take St. John's Wort concurrently with paroxetine.

 NCLEX® Connection: Pharmacological and Parenteral Therapies, Adverse Effects/ Contraindications/Side Effects/Interactions

4. Which of the following interventions is the highest priority regarding management of this client's care?

   A. Placing the client on one-to-one observation

   B. Assisting the client to perform morning care

   C. Encouraging the client to participate in unit activities

   D. Teaching the client about medication side effects

   The greatest risk to this client is injury due to self-harm. Therefore, the highest priority intervention is placing the client on one-to-one observation. Assisting her to perform morning care, encouraging her to participate in unit activities, and teaching her about medication side effects are all important interventions, but they are not the highest priority.

   Ⓝ NCLEX® Connection: Psychosocial Integrity, Crisis Intervention

5. A nurse is interviewing a 25-year-old client diagnosed with dysthymia. Which of the following findings should the nurse expect?

   A. There are wide fluctuations in mood.

   B. There is no evidence of suicidal ideation.

   C. The symptoms last for at least 2 years.

   D. There is an inflated sense of self-esteem.

   Symptoms of dysthymia persist for at least 2 years in adults. Wide fluctuations in mood occur with bipolar disorders, but not with dysthymia. Suicidal ideation may occur in clients with dysthymia. A decreased, rather than inflated, sense of self-esteem is associated with dysthymia.

   Ⓝ NCLEX® Connection: Psychosocial Integrity, Mental Health Concepts

UNIT 3	PSYCHOBIOLOGIC DISORDERS
Chapter 13	Bipolar Disorders

Overview

- Bipolar disorders are mood disorders with recurrent episodes of depression and mania.

- Bipolar disorders usually emerge in late adolescence/early adulthood but can be diagnosed in the school-age child, as well. Because the side effects of medication and bipolar disorder symptoms can mimic the symptoms of Attention Deficit Hyperactivity Disorder (ADHD), children are not usually diagnosed until after the age of seven.

- Periods of normal functioning alternate with periods of illness, though some clients are not able to maintain full occupational and social functioning.

- Psychotic, paranoid, and/or bizarre behavior may be seen during periods of mania.

- Care of a client with bipolar disorder will mirror the phase of the disease that the client is experiencing:

PHASE	CHARACTERISTICS	TREATMENT
Acute	Acute mania	• Treatment is generally 6 to 12 weeks in duration. • Hospitalization may be required. • Reduction of mania symptoms is the goal of treatment. • Risk of harm to self or others is determined. • One-to-one supervision may be indicated.
Maintenance	Increased ability to function	• Treatment is generally 4 to 9 months in duration. • Relapse prevention through education, medication therapy, and psychotherapy is the goal of treatment.
Continuation	Remission of symptoms	• Treatment generally continues throughout the client's lifetime. • Prevention of future manic episodes is the goal of treatment.

- Behaviors shown with bipolar disorders include:

  o Mania – an abnormally elevated mood, which may also be described as expansive or irritable; usually requires inpatient treatment. (See the assessment section in this chapter for specific symptoms.)

  o Hypomania – a less severe episode of mania that lasts at least 4 days accompanied by three to four symptoms of mania. Hospitalization, however, is not required, and the client with hypomania is less impaired.

- ○ Mixed episode – a manic episode and an episode of major depression experienced by the client simultaneously. The client has marked impairment in functioning and may require admission to an acute care mental health facility to prevent self-harm or other-directed violence.

  ○ Rapid cycling – four or more episodes of acute mania within 1 year.

- The various depressive disorders recognized and defined by the DSM-IV-TR include the following:

  ○ Bipolar I disorder – The client has at least one episode of mania alternating with major depression.

  ○ Bipolar II disorder – The client has one or more hypomanic episodes alternating with major depressive episodes.

  ○ Cyclothymia – The client has at least 2 years of repeated hypomanic episodes alternating with minor depressive episodes.

- The following comorbidities are associated with bipolar disorder:

  ○ Substance abuse

    ■ The client with substance abuse issues tends to experience more rapid cycling of mania than do clients who are not abusing.

    ■ Substance use is often use as a means of self-medication. It can have a direct impact on the onset of a mental health disorder, especially if a client is predisposed.

  ○ Anxiety disorders

  ○ Eating disorders

  ○ Attention deficit hyperactivity disorder (ADHD)

Assessment

- Risk Factors

  ○ Physical illness, such as delirium due to a head injury

  ○ Substance abuse, such as cocaine or methamphetamine overdose

- Relapse

  ○ Use of substances (alcohol, drugs of abuse, caffeine) can lead to an episode of mania.

  ○ Sleep disturbances may come before, be associated with, or be brought on by an episode of mania.

- Subjective and Objective Data

BIPOLAR DISORDER SIGNS AND SYMPTOMS	
MANIC CHARACTERISTICS	DEPRESSIVE CHARACTERISTICS
<ul><li>Persistent elevated mood (euphoria)</li><li>Agitation and irritability</li><li>Dislike of interference and intolerance of criticism</li><li>Increase in talking and activities</li><li>Flight of ideas – rapid, continuous speech with sudden and frequent topic change</li><li>Grandiose view of self and abilities (grandiosity)</li><li>Impulsivity: spending money, giving away money or possessions</li><li>Demanding and manipulative behavior</li><li>Distractibility</li><li>Poor judgment</li><li>Attention-seeking behavior: flashy dress and makeup, inappropriate behavior</li><li>Impairment in social and occupational functioning</li><li>Decreased sleep</li><li>Neglect of ADLs, including nutrition and hydration</li><li>Possible presence of delusions and hallucinations</li><li>Denial of illness</li></ul>	<ul><li>Flat, blunted, labile affect</li><li>Tearfulness, crying</li><li>Lack of energy</li><li>Anhedonia: loss of pleasure and lack of interest in activities, hobbies, sexual activity</li><li>Physical symptoms of discomfort/pain</li><li>Difficulty concentrating, focusing, problem solving</li><li>Self-destructive behavior</li><li>Decrease in personal hygiene</li><li>Loss or increase in appetite and/or sleep, disturbed sleep</li><li>Psychomotor retardation or agitation</li></ul>

- Standardized Screening Tool

    ○ Mood Disorders Questionnaire

        ▪ The Mood Disorders Questionnaire is a standardized tool that places mood progression on a continuum for hypomania (euphoria) to acute mania (extreme irritability and hyperactivity) to delirium (completely out of touch with reality).

Collaborative Care

- Nursing Care

  - The care of the client with bipolar disorder will be based on the phase of mania the client is experiencing. Nursing care is provided throughout this process.

  - Acute Phase

    - Focus is on safety and maintaining physical health.

    - Therapeutic Milieu (within acute care mental health facility)

      - Provide a safe environment during the acute phase.

      - Assess the client regularly for suicidal thoughts, intentions, and escalating behavior.

      - Decrease stimulation without isolating the client if possible. Be aware of noise, music, television, and other clients, all of which may lead to an escalation of the client's behavior. In certain cases, seclusion may be the only way to safely decrease stimulation for this client.

      - Follow agency protocols for providing client protection (restraints, seclusion, one-to-one observation) if a threat of self-injury or injury to others exists.

      - Implement frequent rest periods.

      - Observe the client closely for escalating behavior.

      - Provide outlets for physical activity. Do not involve the client in activities that last a long time or that require a high level of concentration and/or detailed instructions.

      - Maintenance of self-care needs includes:

        - Monitoring sleep, fluid intake, and nutrition.

        - Providing portable, nutritious food, since the client may not be able to sit down to eat.

        - Supervising choice of clothes.

        - Giving step-by-step reminders for hygiene and dress.

      - Communication

        - Use a calm, matter-of-fact, specific approach.

        - Give concise explanations.

        - Provide for consistency among staff members.

        - Avoid power struggles, and do not react personally to the client's comments.

        - Listen to and act on legitimate client grievances.

        - Reinforce nonmanipulative behaviors.

- Medications
  - Mood stabilizers
    - Lithium carbonate (Eskalith)
    - Antiepileptic agents that act as mood stabilizers, including: valproic acid (Depakote), clonazepam (Klonopin), lamotrigine (Lamictal), gabapentin (Neurontin), and topiramate (Topax)
  - Benzodiazepines, such as lorazepam (Ativan), used on a short-term basis for a client experiencing sleep impairment related to mania.
  - Antidepressants, such as the SSRI fluoxetine (Prozac), used to manage a major depressive episode
- Therapeutic Procedures
  - Electroconvulsive therapy (ECT)
    - Electroconvulsive therapy (ECT) may be used to subdue extreme manic behavior, especially when pharmacologic therapy, such as lithium, has not worked. ECT may also be used for clients who are suicidal or those with rapid cycling.
- Client Education
  - Case management to provide follow up for the client the family
  - Group, family, and individual psychotherapy to improve problem-solving and interpersonal skills
  - Health teaching regarding:
    - The chronicity of the disorder requiring long-term pharmacological and psychological support
    - Indications of impending relapse and ways to manage the crisis
    - Precipitating factors of relapse (e.g., sleep disturbance, use of alcohol, caffeine, or drugs of abuse)
    - The importance of maintaining a regular sleep, meal, and activity pattern
    - Medication administration
- Client Outcomes
  - The client will refrain from self-harm.
  - The client will rest 4 to 6 hr per night.
  - The client will maintain adequate fluid and food intake.
  - The client will use appropriate communication skills to meet needs.
  - The client will participate in self-care.
  - The client will not experience relapse.

Complications

- Physical Exhaustion and Possible Death
  - A client in a true manic state usually will not stop moving and does not eat, drink, or sleep. This can become a medical emergency.
  - Nursing Actions
    - Prevent client self-harm.
    - Decrease client's physical activity.
    - Promote adequate fluid and food intake.
    - Ensure a minimum of 4 to 6 hr of sleep each night.
    - Assist the client with self-care needs.
    - Manage medication appropriately.

CHAPTER 13: BIPOLAR DISORDERS

 Application Exercises

Scenario: A client in the manic phase of bipolar disorder is being admitted to an inpatient acute care mental health unit. The provider's plan is for this client to undergo a short course of electroconvulsive therapy (ECT) treatments in the first week of hospitalization. The client has been on the unit several times in the past, and his behavior has typically caused upheaval. The staff is verbalizing concerns about the client even before his arrival.

1. List communication principles that the nurse manager should review with the staff regarding this client.

2. Why is ECT used for a client with bipolar disorder?

3. After 1 week on the acute care mental health unit, the client's mania has decreased. However, he has slept very little in the past month. What nursing interventions could assist the client to rest and sleep?

4. A client with mania is standing with a group of clients on the mental health unit. The client is talking excitedly and at great length about a variety of topics. The nurse can see that the other clients are becoming anxious and restless but do not know what to do to stop the conversation. Which of the following is an appropriate response by the nurse?

    A. Tell the client his behavior is annoying others.

    B. Joke to the client that the other clients will collapse if he does not leave them alone.

    C. Tell the client he must leave other clients alone.

    D. Ask the client to come to the dining room for a snack.

CHAPTER 13: BIPOLAR DISORDERS

 Application Exercises Answer Key

Scenario: A client in the manic phase of bipolar disorder is being admitted to an inpatient acute care mental health unit. The provider's plan is for this client to undergo a short course of electroconvulsive therapy (ECT) treatments in the first week of hospitalization. The client has been on the unit several times in the past, and his behavior has typically caused upheaval. The staff is verbalizing concerns about the client even before the client's arrival.

1. List communication principles that the nurse manager should review with the staff regarding this client.

> **Use a firm, calm approach.**
> **Explain things in a short, concise manner.**
> **Refrain from responding personally to the client's comments.**
> **Be consistent in approach and expectations.**
> **Talk with other staff members about what techniques work and do not work.**
> **Adhere to agreed-upon limits.**
> **Let the client know the consequences of inappropriate behavior.**
> **Hear and act on legitimate grievances.**

 NCLEX® Connection: Psychosocial Integrity, Therapeutic Communications

2. Why is ECT used for a client with bipolar disorder?

> **ECT can calm extreme mania in clients with rapid cycling, or if mood stabilizers, such as lithium, fail to provide adequate improvement.**

 NCLEX® Connection: Reduction of Risk Potential, Potential for Complications of Diagnostic Tests/Treatments/Procedures

3. After 1 week on the acute care mental health unit, the client's mania has decreased somewhat. However, he has slept very little in the past month. What nursing interventions could assist this client to rest and sleep?

> **Monitor the client's sleep-wake patterns during the manic phase.**
> **Ascertain the client's normal bedtime routine, such as reading before bedtime, and attempt to facilitate normal patterns as much as possible.**
> **Maintain a quiet, nonstimulating environment in the client's sleeping area.**
> **Limit daytime sleep, if possible, and gradually encourage a return to normal cyclic wake-sleep patterns.**
> **Restrict use of coffee, tea, chocolate, and other stimulants, especially before bedtime.**

NCLEX® Connection: Psychosocial Integrity, Therapeutic Environment

4. A client who is in the manic phase of bipolar disorder is standing with a group of clients on the mental health unit. The client is talking excitedly and at great length about a variety of topics. The nurse can see that the other clients are becoming anxious and restless. Which of the following is an appropriate response by the nurse?

> A. Tell the client his behavior is annoying others.
>
> B. Joke to the client that the other clients will collapse if he does not leave them alone.
>
> C. Tell the client he must leave other clients alone.
>
> **D. Ask the client to come to the dining room for a snack.**
>
> A client who is in the manic phase of bipolar disorder is easily distracted, and this can be a good technique for directing him to more appropriate activities without causing a power struggle. The other techniques would likely cause anger, or at least argument.

(N) NCLEX® Connection: Psychosocial Integrity, Behavioral Interventions

UNIT 3	PSYCHOBIOLOGIC DISORDERS
Chapter 14	Schizophrenia

Overview

- Schizophrenia is a group of psychotic disorders that affect thinking, behavior, emotions, and the ability to perceive reality.

- Schizophrenia probably results from a combination of genetic and nongenetic factors (injury at birth, nutritional factors, viral infection, and hormonal imbalances).

- The typical age at onset is late teens and early twenties, but schizophrenia has occurred in young children and may begin in later adulthood.

- A diagnosis of schizophrenia should not be made for children until after age 7 to rule out attention deficit hyperactivity disorder (ADHD) with violent tendencies.

- Schizophrenia becomes problematic when symptoms interfere with interpersonal relationships, self-care, and ability to work.

- Categories/Taxonomies of Disorder

  o The various types of schizophrenia recognized and defined by the DSM-IV-TR include:

TYPE OF SCHIZOPHRENIA	COMMON SYMPTOMS
Paranoid • Characterized by suspicion toward others.	• Hallucinations, such as hearing threatening voices, and delusions, such as believing oneself president of the United States • Other-directed violence may occur.
Disorganized • Characterized by withdrawal from society and very inappropriate behaviors, such as poor hygiene or muttering constantly to oneself. • Frequently seen in the homeless population.	• Loose associations • Bizarre mannerisms • Incoherent speech • Hallucinations and delusions may be present but are much less organized than those seen in the client with paranoia.

TYPE OF SCHIZOPHRENIA	COMMON SYMPTOMS
Catatonic • Characterized by abnormal motor movements. • There are two stages: the withdrawn stage and the excited stage.	Withdrawn stage • Psychomotor retardation; the client may appear comatose. • Waxy flexibility may be present. • The client often has extreme self-care needs, such as for tube feeding due to an inability to eat. Excited stage • Constant movement, unusual posturing, incoherent speech • Self-care needs may predominate. • The client may be a danger to self or others.
Residual • Active symptoms are no longer present, but the client has two or more "residual" symptoms.	• Anergia, anhedonia, or avolition • Withdrawal from social activities • Impaired role function • Speech problems, such as alogia • Odd behaviors, such as walking in a strange way
Undifferentiated • The client has symptoms of schizophrenia but does not meet criteria for any of the other types.	• Any positive or negative symptoms may be present.

- Other psychotic disorders include:

  o Schizoaffective disorder – The client's disorder meets both the criteria for schizophrenia and one of the affective disorders (depression, mania, or a mixed disorder).

  o Brief psychotic disorder – The client has psychotic symptoms that last between 1 day to 1 month in duration.

  o Schizophreniform disorder – The client has symptoms like those of schizophrenia, but the duration is from 1 to 6 months and social/occupational dysfunction may or may not be present.

  o Shared psychotic disorder – One person begins to share the delusional beliefs of another person with psychosis. This is also called *Folie à Deux*.

  o Secondary (induced) psychosis – Signs of psychosis are brought on by a medical disorder, such as Alzheimer's disease, or by use of chemical substances, such as alcohol abuse.

Assessment

- Subjective and Objective Data

CHARACTERISTIC DIMENSIONS OF SCHIZOPHRENIA	
CHARACTERISTICS	EXAMPLES OF BEHAVIOR IN EACH DIMENSION
Positive symptoms – These are the most easily identified symptoms.	• Hallucinations • Delusions • Alterations in speech • Bizarre behavior, such as walking backward constantly
Negative symptoms – These symptoms are more difficult to treat successfully than positive symptoms.	• Affect – usually blunted (narrow range of normal expression) or flat (facial expression never changes) • Alogia – poverty of thought or speech; the client may sit with a visitor but may only mumble or respond vaguely to questions. • Avolition – lack of motivation in activities and hygiene; for example, the client completes an assigned task, such as making his bed, but is unable to start the next common chore without prompting. • Anhedonia – lack of pleasure or joy; the client is indifferent to things that often make others happy, such as looking at beautiful scenery. • Anergia – lack of energy

Cognitive symptoms – Problems with thinking make it very difficult for the client to live independently.	• Disordered thinking
	• Inability to make decisions
	• Poor problem-solving ability
	• Difficulty concentrating to perform tasks
	• Memory deficits
	  ◦ Long-term memory
	  ◦ Working memory, such as inability to follow directions to find an address

Depressive symptoms	• Hopelessness • Suicidal ideation

○ Alterations in thought (delusions) are false fixed beliefs that cannot be corrected by reasoning and are usually bizarre. These include:

DELUSIONS	EXAMPLES
Ideas of reference	Misconstrues trivial events and attaches personal significance to them, such as believing that others, who are discussing the next meal, are talking about him.
Persecution	Feels singled out for harm by others (e.g., being hunted down by the FBI).
Grandeur	Believes that she is all powerful and important, like a god.
Somatic delusions	Believes that his body is changing in an unusual way, such as growing a third arm.
Jealousy	May feel that her spouse is sexually involved with another individual.
Being controlled	Believes that a force outside his body is controlling him.
Thought broadcasting	Believes that her thoughts are heard by others.
Thought insertion	Believes that others' thoughts are being inserted into his mind.
Thought withdrawal	Believes that her thoughts have been removed from her mind by an outside agency.
Religiosity	Is obsessed with religious beliefs.

○ Following are examples of alterations in speech that can occur with schizophrenia:

ALTERATIONS IN SPEECH	
Flight of ideas	• Associative looseness • The client may say sentence after sentence, but each sentence may relate to another topic, and the listener is unable to follow the client's thoughts.
Neologisms	• Made up words that only have meaning to the client, such as, "I tranged and flittled."
Echolalia	• The client repeats the words spoken to him.
Clang association	• Meaningless rhyming of words, often forceful, such as, "Oh fox, box, and lox."
Word salad	• Words jumbled together with little meaning or significance to listener, such as, "Hip hooray, the flip is cast and wide-sprinting in the forest."

○ Alterations in perception

■ Hallucinations are sensory perceptions that do not have any apparent external stimulus. Examples include:

□ Auditory – hearing voices or sounds that may take the form of commands instructing the client to hurt self or others.

□ Visual – seeing persons or things.

□ Olfactory – smelling odors.

□ Gustatory – experiencing tastes.

□ Tactile – feeling bodily sensations.

- Personal boundary difficulties – disenfranchisement with one's own body, identity, and perceptions. This includes:

  □ Depersonalization – nonspecific feeling that a person has lost her identity; self is different or unreal.

  □ Derealization – perception that environment has changed.

- Alterations in behavior

  □ Extreme agitation, including pacing and rocking

  □ Stereotyped behaviors – motor patterns that had meaning to client (sweeping the floor) but now are mechanical and lack purpose

  □ Automatic obedience – responding in a robot-like manner

  □ Wavy flexibility – excessive maintenance of position

  □ Stupor – motionless for long periods of time, coma-like

  □ Negativism – doing the opposite of what is requested

  □ Echopraxia – purposeful imitation of movements made by others

- Standardized Screening Tools

  ○ The Global Assessment of Functioning (GAF) scale – helps to determine a client's ability to perform activities of daily living and to function independently

  ○ Scale for Assessment of Negative Symptoms

  ○ Simpson Neurological Rating Scale

Collaborative Care

- Nursing Care

  ○ Milieu therapy is utilized for clients with schizophrenia both in 24-hr mental health facilities and in community facilities, such as adult day care programs.

    - Provide a structured, safe environment (milieu) for the client in order to decrease anxiety and to distract the client from constant thinking about hallucinations.

  ○ Promote therapeutic communication to lower anxiety, decrease defensive patterns, and encourage participation in the milieu.

  ○ Establish a trusting relationship with the client.

  ○ Encourage the development of social skills and friendships.

  ○ Encourage participation in group work and psychotherapy.

o   Use appropriate communication to address hallucinations and delusions.

- Ask the client directly about hallucinations. The nurse should not argue or agree with client's view of the situation, but may offer a comment, such as, "I don't hear anything, but you seem to be feeling frightened."

- Do not argue with a client's delusions, but focus on the client's feelings and possibly offer reasonable explanations, such as, "I can't imagine that the President of the United States would have a reason to kill a citizen, but it must be frightening for you to believe that."

- Provide for safety if the client is experiencing command hallucinations.

- Attempt to focus conversations on reality-based subjects.

- Identify symptom triggers, such as loud noises (may trigger auditory hallucinations in certain clients) and situations that seem to trigger conversations about the client's delusions.

- Be genuine and empathetic in all dealings with the client.

o   Assess discharge needs, such as ability to perform activities of daily living.

o   Promote self-care by modeling and teaching self-care activities within the mental health facility.

o   Relate wellness to the elements of symptom management.

o   Collaborate with the client to use symptom management techniques to cope with depressive symptoms and anxiety. Symptom management techniques include such strategies as using music to distract from "voices," attending activities, walking, talking to a trusted person when hallucinations are most bothersome, and interacting with an auditory or visual hallucination by telling it to stop or go away.

o   Encourage medication compliance.

o   Provide teaching regarding medications.

TEACHING	EXAMPLES OF MEDICATION	USES FOR MEDICATION
Atypical antipsychotics are current medications of choice for psychotic disorders, and they generally treat both positive and negative symptoms.	• Risperidone (Risperdal) • Olanzapine (Zyprexa) • Quetiapine (Seroquel) • Ziprasidone (Geodon) • Aripiprazole (Abilify) • Clozapine (Clozaril)	• To minimize weight gain advise the client to follow a healthy, low-calorie diet, engage in regular exercise, and monitor weight gain. • Symptoms of agitation, dizziness, sedation, and sleep disruption may occur. Instruct the client to report these side effects to his provider, as the medication may need to be changed.

TEACHING	EXAMPLES OF MEDICATION	USES FOR MEDICATION
Conventional antipsychotics are used to treat mainly positive psychotic symptoms.	• Haloperidol (Haldol) • Loxapine (Loxitane) • Chlorpromazine (Thorazine) • Fluphenazine (Prolixin)	• To minimize anticholinergic effects, advise the client to chew sugarless gum, eat foods high in fiber, and to eat and drink 2 to 3 L of fluid/day from food and beverage sources. • Instruct the client about signs of postural hypotension (e.g., light-headedness, dizziness). If these occur, advise the client to sit or lie down. Orthostatic hypotension can be minimized by getting up slowly from a lying or sitting position.
Antidepressants are used to treat the depression seen in many clients with schizophrenia.	Paroxetine (Paxil)	• Used temporarily to treat depression associated with schizophrenia. • Monitor the client for suicidal ideation, as this medication may increase thoughts of self-harm, especially when first taking it. • Notify the provider of any side effects, such as deepened depression. • Advise client to avoid abrupt cessation of this medication to avoid a withdrawal effect.
Anxiolytics/benzodiazepines are used to treat the anxiety often found in clients with schizophrenia, as well as some of the positive and negative symptoms of schizophrenia.	• Lorazepam (Ativan) • Clonazepam (Klonopin)	• Inform the client of this medication's sedative effects. • Inform the client the need for blood tests to monitor for agranulocytosis. • These medications are used with caution in older adult clients.

- Care After Discharge

  - Client Education

    - Case management to provide follow up for the client and family

    - Group, family, and individual psychotherapy to improve problem-solving and interpersonal skills

    - Health teaching regarding the following:

      - Need for self-care to prevent relapse

      - Medication effects, side effects, and importance of compliance

      - Importance of attending support groups

      - Abstinence from the use of alcohol and/or drugs

      - Keeping a log or journal of feelings and changes in behavior to help monitor medication effectiveness

- Client Outcomes

  - The client will regularly attend support groups.

  - The client will maintain an appropriate level of self-care.

  - The client will maintain medication adherence.

CHAPTER 14: SCHIZOPHRENIA

 Application Exercises

1. A 19-year-old college student comes to a mental health emergency facility experiencing hallucinations. Describe strategies for working with this client and lessening the effects of her hallucinations.

2. Positive symptoms of schizophrenia include which of the following? (Select all that apply.)

_____ Auditory hallucination

_____ Lack of motivation

_____ Use of clang associations

_____ Delusion of persecution

_____ Motor agitation

_____ Flat affect

3. A client with schizophrenia has great difficulty with personal boundaries. Which of the following is a personal boundary problem?

    A. Delusions of grandeur or persecution

    B. Depersonalization or derealization

    C. Visual or auditory hallucinations

    D. Communication difficulties or social withdrawal

4. A nurse is speaking with a client who has schizophrenia when he suddenly seems to stop focusing on the nurse's questions and begins looking at the ceiling and talking to himself. Which of the following actions should the nurse take?

    A. Stop the interview at this point and resume later when the client is better able to concentrate.

    B. Ask the client, "Are you seeing something on the ceiling?"

    C. Tell the client, "You seem to be looking at something on the ceiling. I see something there, too."

    D. Continue the interview without comment on the client's behavior.

5. Which of the following are associated with catatonic schizophrenia?

    A. Purposeless motor agitations

    B. Tactile hallucinations

    C. Word salad and flight of ideas

    D. Eccentric behaviors or odd beliefs

6. Match the symptoms below with the appropriate psychotic disorders.

_____ Schizophreniform disorder

_____ Schizoaffective disorder

_____ Shared psychotic disorder

_____ Brief psychotic disorder

_____ Induced psychosis

A. Psychotic symptoms caused by abuse of chemical substances or physical illness

B. An episode of psychotic behavior lasting from 1 day to 1 month in length

C. Psychotic behavior lasting between 1 and 6 months that may not impair the client's ability to function at work or in social occasions

D. Symptoms of schizophrenia along with symptoms of mania or major depression

E. One person sharing the delusional beliefs of another person with psychosis

7. A nurse is caring for a client on an inpatient mental health unit. The client reports hearing voices that are telling her to "kill your roommate." Which of the following actions should the nurse take?

A. Tell the client that she is imagining the voices.

B. Initiate one-to-one observation of the client.

C. Place the client in a restraint.

D. Ask another client to sit with the client.

CHAPTER 14: SCHIZOPHRENIA

 Application Exercises Answer Key

1. A 19-year-old college student comes to a mental health emergency facility experiencing hallucinations. Describe strategies for working with this client and lessening the effects of her hallucinations.

> Establish a trusting nurse-client relationship.
> Assess for characteristics of hallucinations, including duration, intensity, frequency, and type.
> Focus on the symptom – the "feelings" – and ask the client to describe what is happening.
> Identify whether drugs or alcohol have been used.
> If asked, point out that you are not experiencing the same stimuli.
> Help the client describe and compare current and past hallucinations.
> Help the client identify needs that may be reflected in the content of the hallucinations.
> Determine the impact of the client's symptoms on ADLs.

 NCLEX® Connection: Psychosocial Integrity, Mental Health Concepts

2. Positive symptoms of schizophrenia include which of the following? (Select all that apply.)

__X__	**Auditory hallucination**
_____	Lack of motivation
__X__	**Use of clang associations**
__X__	**Delusion of persecution**
__X__	**Motor agitation**
_____	Flat affect

> Auditory hallucinations, use of clang associations, delusions of persecution, and motor agitation are all positive symptoms of schizophrenia. Lack of motivation (or avolition) and flat affect (facial expression) are negative symptoms.

 NCLEX® Connection: Psychosocial Integrity, Mental Health Concepts

3. A client with schizophrenia has great difficulty with personal boundaries. Which of the following is a personal boundary problem?

> A. Delusions of grandeur or persecution
>
> **B. Depersonalization or derealization**
>
> C. Visual or auditory hallucinations
>
> D Communication difficulties or social withdrawal

> Depersonalization (a feeling of being separated from one's body) and derealization (a sensation of being in a strange environment) are examples of problems with personal boundaries. Delusions and hallucinations are positive symptoms of schizophrenia. Problems with communication or social withdrawal may be present in schizophrenia, but they are not personal boundary issues.

 NCLEX® Connection: Psychosocial Integrity, Mental Health Concepts

4. A nurse is speaking with a client who has schizophrenia when he suddenly seems to stop focusing on the nurse's questions and begins looking at the ceiling and talking to himself. Which of the following actions should the nurse take?

A. Stop the interview at this point and resume later when the client is better able to concentrate.

B. Ask the client, "Are you seeing something on the ceiling?"

C. Tell the client, "You seem to be looking at something on the ceiling. I see something there, too."

D. Continue the interview without comment on the client's behavior.

The appropriate action for the nurse to take is to ask the client directly about his hallucinations, but avoid treating hallucinations or delusions as if they were real. Stopping the interview until a later time may not be feasible since the client may experience hallucinations much of the time. Continuing the interview without commenting on this client's hallucinations will not be an effective distraction.

(N) **NCLEX® Connection: Psychosocial Integrity, Behavioral Interventions**

5. Which of the following are associated with catatonic schizophrenia?

A. Purposeless motor agitations

B. Tactile hallucinations

C. Word salad and flight of ideas

D. Eccentric behaviors or odd beliefs

Purposeless motor agitation or activity are characteristics of the excited phase of catatonic schizophrenia. Hallucinations are seen in clients with paranoid, disorganized, and undifferentiated types of schizophrenia. Word salad and flight of ideas are communication abnormalities seen in other types of schizophrenia. Eccentric behavior and odd beliefs are found in clients with residual schizophrenia.

(N) **NCLEX® Connection: Psychosocial Integrity, Mental Health Concepts**

6. Match the symptoms below with the appropriate psychotic disorders.

__C__	Schizophreniform disorder	A. Psychotic symptoms caused by abuse of chemical substances or physical illness
__D__	Schizoaffective disorder	B. An episode of psychotic behavior lasting from 1 day to 1 month in length
__E__	Shared psychotic disorder	C. Psychotic behavior lasting between 1 and 6 months that may not impair the client's ability to function at work or in social occasions
__B__	Brief psychotic disorder	D. Symptoms of schizophrenia along with symptoms of mania or major depression
__A__	Induced psychosis	E. One person sharing the delusional beliefs of another person with psychosis

(N) **NCLEX® Connection: Psychosocial Integrity, Mental Health Concepts**

7. A nurse is caring for a client on an inpatient mental health unit. The client reports hearing voices that are telling her to "kill your roommate." Which of the following actions should the nurse take?

    A. Tell the client that she is imagining the voices.

    B. Initiate one-to-one observation of the client.

    C. Place the client in a restraint.

    D. Ask another client to sit with the client.

The client is at risk for harming someone else or himself and therefore needs to be watched closely. Telling him he is imagining the voices is a nontherapeutic response. It is not appropriate to place this client in a vest restraint. Asking another client to sit with him places that client at risk for harm.

(N) **NCLEX® Connection: Safety and Infection Control, Injury Prevention**

UNIT 3   PSYCHOBIOLOGIC DISORDERS

Chapter 15   Personality Disorders

Overview

- A client with a personality disorder demonstrates long-term maladaptive behavior that prevents accomplishment of desired goals in relationships and other efforts.

- The maladaptive behaviors of a personality disorder are not experienced as uncomfortable by the individual, and some areas of personal functioning may be very adequate.

- Personality disorders are predisposing factors for many other psychiatric disorders and often co-occur with depression and anxiety.

- Personality disorders have a significant effect on the course of treatment for other psychiatric disorders.

- The various personality disorders recognized and defined by the DSM-IV-TR are as follows:

    o Cluster A – generally described as odd or eccentric

    o Cluster B – generally described as dramatic, emotional, or erratic

    o Cluster C – generally described as anxious or fearful

- Defense mechanisms used by clients with personality disorders include repression, suppression, regression, undoing, and splitting.

    o Of these, splitting, which is the inability to incorporate positive and negative aspects of oneself or others into a whole image, is frequently seen in the inpatient setting.

    o Splitting is commonly associated with borderline personality disorder.

    o In splitting, the client tends to characterize people or things as all good or all bad at any particular moment. For example, the client might say, "You are the worst person in the world." Later that day she might say, "You are the best, but the nurse from the last shift is absolutely terrible."

Assessment

- Risk Factors

    o Individuals with personality disorders tend to be less educated or unemployed; are single or have marital difficulties; often have comorbid substance use disorders, and may commit nonviolent and violent crimes, including sex offenses.

- o Environmental influences – such as child abuse, biological influences (genetic factors), and psychological factors – appear to play a role in the etiology of personality disorders.
- Subjective and Objective Data
  - o All personality disorders share four common characteristics:
    - Inflexibility/maladaptive responses to stress
    - Disability in social and professional relationships
    - Tendency to provoke interpersonal conflict
    - Ability to merge personal boundaries with others

THE 10 PERSONALITY DISORDERS		
Cluster A (Odd or eccentric traits)	Paranoid	Characterized by distrust and suspiciousness toward others based on unfounded beliefs that others want to harm, exploit, or deceive the person
	Schizoid	Characterized by emotional detachment, disinterest in close relationships, and indifference to praise or criticism; often uncooperative
	Schizotypal	Characterized by odd beliefs leading to interpersonal difficulties, an eccentric appearance, and magical thinking or perceptual distortions that are not clear delusions or hallucinations
Cluster B (Dramatic, emotional, or erratic traits)	Antisocial	Characterized by disregard for others with exploitation, repeated unlawful actions, deceit, and failure to accept personal responsibility
	Borderline	Characterized by instability of affect, identity, and relationships; fear of abandonment, splitting behaviors, manipulation, and impulsiveness; often tries self-mutilation and may be suicidal
	Histrionic	Characterized by emotional attention-seeking behavior, in which the person needs to be the center of attention; often seductive and flirtatious
	Narcissistic	Characterized by arrogance, grandiose views of self-importance, the need for consistent admiration, and a lack of empathy for others that strains most relationships; often sensitive to criticism

THE 10 PERSONALITY DISORDERS		
Cluster C (Anxious or fearful traits; insecurity and inadequacy)	Avoidant	Characterized by social inhibition and avoidance of all situations that require interpersonal contact, despite wanting close relationships, due to extreme fear of rejection; often very anxious in social situations
	Dependent	Characterized by extreme dependency in a close relationship with an urgent search to find a replacement when one relationship ends; the most frequently-seen personality disorder in the clinical setting
	Obsessive compulsive	Characterized by perfectionism with a focus on orderliness and control to the extent that the individual may not be able to accomplish a given task

Collaborative Care

- Nursing Care

  ○ Self-assessment is vital for nurses caring for clients with personality disorders; clients with personality disorders may evoke intense feelings in the nurse.

  ○ Milieu therapy in a group context is aimed at the specific personality disorder.

  ○ Safety is always a priority concern, since some clients with a personality disorder are at risk for self- or other-directed violence.

  ○ Communication strategies

    ▪ Developing a therapeutic relationship is often challenging due to the client's distrust or hostility toward others. Feelings of being threatened or having no control may cause a client to act out toward the nurse.

      □ A firm, yet supportive approach and consistent care will help build a therapeutic nurse-client relationship.

      □ Offer the client realistic choices to enhance the client's sense of control.

      □ Limit-setting and consistency are essential with clients who are manipulative, especially those with borderline or antisocial personality disorders.

      □ Assertiveness training and modeling can be important for clients with dependent and histrionic personality disorders.

      □ For clients with histrionic personality disorder, who may be very flirtatious, it is important to maintain professional boundaries and communication.

      □ Clients with schizoid or schizotypal personality disorders tend to isolate themselves, and this need for social isolation should be respected.

      □ For very dependent clients, self-assess frequently for countertransference reactions to the client's clinging and frequent requests for help.

- Medications

  o Medications include the use of psychotropic agents that are geared toward maintaining cognitive function and relieving symptoms. Antidepressant, anxiolytic, antipsychotic, or a combination of these medications may be prescribed.

- Interdisciplinary Care

  o Psychobiological interventions include the following:

    ▪ Dialectical behavior therapy is a cognitive-behavioral therapy used for clients with borderline personality disorder. It focuses on gradual behavior changes and provides acceptance and validation for these clients, who are very frequently (80% of cases) suicidal and have self-mutilating behaviors.

    ▪ Case management is beneficial for clients who have personality disorders and are persistently and severely impaired.

      ☐ In acute care facilities, case management focuses on obtaining pertinent history from current or previous providers, supporting reintegration with the family, and ensuring appropriate referrals to outpatient care.

      ☐ In long-term outpatient facilities, case management goals include reducing hospitalization by providing resources for crisis services and enhancing the social support system.

CHAPTER 15: PERSONALITY DISORDERS

(A) Application Exercises

Scenario: A nurse on an inpatient psychiatric unit is asked to conduct a staff inservice about communicating with clients who have personality disorders. The nursing staff includes registered nurses, licensed practical nurses, and mental health technicians. Although some of them have previous mental health work experience, none of them has worked in a mental health facility for more than 5 years, and there is disagreement among the staff about the best strategies for caring for clients who have personality disorders.

1. Identify three components of care that are important to include in the inservice.

2. What communication strategies should the nurse suggest using with clients who have personality disorders?

3. Match the letter of the description with the personality disorder to which it corresponds.

_____ Borderline

_____ Antisocial

_____ Obsessive compulsive

_____ Histrionic

_____ Avoidant

_____ Schizoid

A. Perfectionistic and orderly, demands control of every situation

B. Evades all social situations and fears rejection

C. Emotionally detached and disinterested in others; uninterested in praise or criticism

D. Deceitful, manipulative, and unlawful, does not take responsibility for actions

E. Emotional with unstable identity and relationships; fears abandonment but uses splitting, which angers others

F. Needs to be the center of attention in all situations

4. A nurse has denied a request from a client with borderline personality disorder. The client says, "The nurse on the evening shift would never be nasty to me like you are! You are a horrible, awful person!" This is an example of

A. regression.

B. splitting.

C. undoing.

D. identification.

5. A client with antisocial personality disorder is admitted to a chemical dependency unit. The nurse should expect which of the following behaviors? (Select all that apply.)

_____ Anxious

_____ Indecisive

_____ Exploitative

_____ Submissive

_____ Aggressive

_____ Impulsive

CHAPTER 15: PERSONALITY DISORDERS

 Application Exercises Answer Key

Scenario: A nurse on an inpatient psychiatric unit is asked to conduct a staff inservice about communicating with clients who have personality disorders. The nursing staff includes registered nurses, licensed practical nurses, and mental health technicians. Although some of them have previous mental health work experience, none of them has worked in a mental health facility for more than 5 years, and there is disagreement among the staff about the best strategies for caring for clients who have personality disorders.

1. Identify three components of care that are important to include in the inservice.

Clients with personality disorders have a tendency to cause frustration and stress in those caring for them. Self-awareness is important when providing care for these clients in order to maintain professionalism and promote the well-being of the client. Effective communication among staff is also important, as many clients with personality disorders use the defense mechanism splitting in an effort to get their needs met. Limit setting is often necessary with clients who have personality disorders. Other important topics to cover should include establishing trust with these clients, keeping the clients safe, and enhancing their involvement and sense of control over their care.

Ⓝ NCLEX® Connection: Psychosocial Integrity, Behavioral Interventions

2. What communication strategies should the nurse suggest using with clients who have personality disorders?

Effective communication strategies when dealing with clients who have personality disorders include utilizing direct, honest communication, limit-setting, and assertiveness.

Ⓝ NCLEX® Connection: Psychosocial Integrity, Therapeutic Communications

3. Match the letter of the description with the personality disorder to which it corresponds.

E	Borderline	A. Perfectionistic and orderly, demands control of every situation
D	Antisocial	B. Evades all social situations and fears rejection
A	Obsessive compulsive	C. Emotionally detached and disinterested in others; uninterested in praise or criticism
F	Histrionic	D. Deceitful, manipulative, and unlawful, does not take responsibility for actions
B	Avoidant	E. Emotional with unstable identity and relationships; fears abandonment but uses splitting, which angers others
C	Schizoid	F. Needs to be the center of attention in all situations

Ⓝ NCLEX® Connection: Psychosocial Integrity, Mental Health Concepts

4. A nurse has denied a request from a client with borderline personality disorder. The client says, "The nurse on the evening shift would never be nasty to me like you are! You are a horrible, awful person!" This is an example of

    A. regression.

    B. splitting.

    C. undoing.

    D. identification.

Splitting occurs when a person is unable to see both positive and negative qualities at the same time. The client with borderline personality disorder tends to see a person as all bad one time and all good another time. Regression refers to resorting to an earlier way of functioning, such as having a temper tantrum. Undoing is a behavior that is intended to undo or reverse unacceptable thoughts or acts, such as buying a gift for a spouse after having lunch with a coworker of the opposite sex. In identification, the person imitates the behavior of someone admired or feared.

 NCLEX® Connection: Psychosocial Integrity, Mental Health Concepts

5. A client with antisocial personality disorder is admitted to a chemical dependency unit. The nurse should expect which of the following behaviors? (Select all that apply.)

    _____ Anxious

    _____ Indecisive

    __X__ **Exploitative**

    _____ Submissive

    __X__ **Aggressive**

    __X__ **Impulsive**

A client with antisocial personality disorder typically displays behaviors that are aggressive, manipulative, exploitative, callous, impulsive, and guilt-instilling. They rarely appear anxious, indecisive, or submissive.

 NCLEX® Connection: Psychosocial Integrity, Mental Health Concepts

UNIT 3	PSYCHOBIOLOGIC DISORDERS
Chapter 16	Cognitive Disorders

Overview

- Cognitive disorders are a group of conditions characterized by the disruption of thinking, memory, processing, and problem solving.

- Treatment of clients with cognitive disorders requires a compassionate understanding of both the client and the family.

- The various cognitive disorders recognized and defined by the DSM-IV-TR include the following:

  o Delirium

  o Dementia

  o Amnestic disorders

Assessment

- Risk Factors

  o Risk factors for cognitive disorders include physiological changes, including neurological (Parkinson's disease, Huntington's disease); metabolic (hepatic or renal failure, fluid and electrolyte imbalances, nutritional deficiencies); and cardiovascular diseases; family genetics; infections (HIV/AIDS); tumors; substance abuse; drug intoxication; and drug withdrawal.

  o Risk factors for Alzheimer's disease include advanced age, female gender, prior head trauma, and a family history of Alzheimer's disease and/or trisomy (Down syndrome).

- Subjective and Objective Data

  o Delirium and dementia have some similarities and some important differences:

	DELIRIUM	DEMENTIA
Onset	Rapid over a short period of time (hours or days)	Gradual deterioration of function over months or years
Signs and symptoms	• Occurrence of impairments in memory, judgment, ability to focus, and ability to calculate; these impairments may fluctuate throughout the day. • Level of consciousness is usually altered. • Restlessness, agitation are common; sundowning (confusion during the night) may occur; behaviors may increase or decrease daily. • Personality change is rapid. • Some perceptual disturbances may be present, such as hallucinations and illusions. • Vital signs may be unstable and abnormal due to medical illness.	• Impairments in memory, judgment, speech (aphasia), ability to recognize familiar objects (agnosia), executive functioning (managing daily tasks), and movement (apraxia); impairments do not change throughout the day. • Level of consciousness is usually unchanged. • Restlessness, agitation are common; sundowning may occur; behaviors usually remain stable. • Personality change is gradual. • Vital signs are stable unless other illness is present.
Cause	• Caused secondary to another medical condition, such as infection, or to substance abuse	• Generally caused by a chronic disease, such as Alzheimer's disease, or is the result of chronic alcohol abuse • May be caused by permanent trauma, such as head injury
Outcome	• Reversible if diagnosis and treatment are prompt	• Irreversible and progressive

STAGES OF ALZHEIMER'S DISEASE (RETRIEVED 4.27.09 FROM WWW.ALZ.ORG)	
STAGE	SIGNS AND SYMPTOMS
Stage 1: No impairment (normal function)	• No memory problems • No memory problems evident to provider
Stage 2: Very mild cognitive decline, which may be normal age-related changes, or very early signs of Alzheimer's disease	• Forgetfulness, especially of everyday objects (eyeglasses, wallet) • No memory problems evident to provider, friends, or coworkers

STAGES OF ALZHEIMER'S DISEASE (RETRIEVED 4.27.09 FROM WWW.ALZ.ORG)	
STAGE	SIGNS AND SYMPTOMS
Stage 3: Mild cognitive decline, including problems with memory or concentration that may be measurable in clinical testing or during a detailed medical interview	• Mild cognitive deficits, including losing or misplacing important objects, decreased ability to plan • Short-term memory loss noticeable to close relations • Decreased attention span • Difficulty remembering words or names • Difficulty in social or work situations
Stage 4: Moderate cognitive decline (mild or early-stage Alzheimer's disease) that is clearly detected during a medical interview	• Personality change: appearing withdrawn or subdued, especially in social or mentally challenging situations • Obvious memory loss • Limited knowledge and memory of recent occasions, current events, or personal history • Difficulty performing tasks that require planning and organizing (paying bills, managing money) • Difficulty with complex mental arithmetic
Stage 5: Moderately severe cognitive decline (moderate or mid-stage Alzheimer's disease)	• Increasing cognitive deficits • Inability to recall important details, such as address and telephone number, but ability to remember information about self and family • Disorientation and confusion as to time and place
Stage 6: Severe cognitive decline (moderately severe or mid-stage Alzheimer's disease)	• Continued worsening of memory difficulties • Loss of awareness of recent events and surroundings • Ability to recall own name but not personal history • Evidence of significant personality changes (delusions, hallucinations, compulsive behaviors) • Wandering behavior • Assistance required for usual daily activities, such as dressing, toileting, and other grooming • Disruption of normal sleep/wake cycle • Increased episodes of urinary and fecal incontinence • Violent tendencies with potential danger to self or others
Stage 7: Very severe cognitive decline (severe or late-stage Alzheimer's disease)	• Loss of ability to respond to environment, to speak, and to control movement • Unrecognizable speech, general urinary incontinence, inability to eat without assistance, and impaired swallowing • Gradual loss of all ability to move • Stupor and coma • Death frequently related to choking or infection

- Defense Mechanisms Used in Cognitive Disorders

  o Assess for defense mechanisms used by the client to preserve self-esteem when cognitive changes are progressive:

    ▪ Denial – Both the client and family members may refuse to believe that changes, such as loss of memory, are taking place, even when those changes are obvious to others.

    ▪ Confabulation – The client may make up stories when questioned about events or activities that she does not remember. This may seem like lying, but it is actually an unconscious attempt to save self-esteem and prevent admitting that she does not remember the occasion.

    ▪ Perseveration – The client avoids answering questions by repeating phrases or behavior. This is another unconscious attempt to maintain self-esteem when memory has failed.

- Amnestic disorder may be secondary to substance abuse or another medical condition. Typically there is no personality change or impairment in abstract thinking. Changes due to amnestic disorder include the following:

  o Decreased awareness of surroundings

  o Inability to learn new information despite normal attention

  o Inability to recall previously learned information

  o Possible disorientation to place and time

- Laboratory and Diagnostic Tests

  o Chest and skull x-rays

  o Electroencephalography (EEG)

  o Electrocardiography (ECG)

  o Liver function studies

  o Thyroid function tests

  o Neuroimaging (computer tomography and position emission tomography of the brain)

  o Urinalysis

  o Serum electrolytes

- Standardized Screening Tools

  o Functional Dementia Scale

    ▪ Use of this tool will give the nurse information regarding the client's ability to perform self-care, the extent of the client's memory loss, mood changes, and the degree of danger to self and/or others.

  o Mini-Mental Status Examination

     ○   Functional Assessment Screening Tool

     ○   Global Deterioration Scale

Collaborative Care

- Nursing Care

  ○ Perform self-assessment regarding possible feelings of frustration, anger, or fear when performing daily care for clients with progressive dementia.

  ○ Nursing interventions are focused on protecting the client from injury, as well as promoting client dignity and quality of life.

  ○ Provide for a safe and therapeutic environment

  - Assign the client to a room close to the nurse's station for close observation.

  - Provide a room with a low level of visual and auditory stimuli.

  - Provide for a well-lit environment, minimizing contrasts and shadows.

  - Have the client sit in a room with windows to help with time orientation.

  - Have the client wear an identification bracelet; use monitors and bed alarm devices as needed.

  - Use restraints only as an intervention of last resort.

  - Administer medications PRN for agitation or anxiety.

  - Ensure safety in the physical environment, such as a lowered bed and removal of scatter rugs to prevent falls.

  - Provide compensatory memory aids, such as clocks, calendars, photographs, memorabilia, seasonal decorations, and familiar objects. Reorient as necessary.

  - Provide eyeglasses and assistive hearing devices as needed.

  - Keep a consistent daily routine.

  - Maintain consistent caregivers.

  - Ensure adequate food and fluid intake.

  - Allow for safe pacing and wandering.

  - Cover or remove mirrors to decrease fear and agitation.

  ○ Communication

  - Communicate in a calm, reassuring tone.

  - Do not argue or question hallucinations or delusions.

  - Reinforce reality.

  - Reinforce orientation to time, place, and person.

  - Introduce self to client with each new contact.

  - Establish eye contact and use short, simple sentences when speaking to the client.

- Encourage reminiscence about happy times; talk about familiar things.
- Break instructions and activities into short timeframes.
- Limit the number of choices when dressing or eating.
- Minimize the need for decision making and abstract thinking to avoid frustration.
- Avoid confrontation.
- Encourage family visitation as appropriate.

- Medications

  ○ Medications, such as donepezil (Aricept), rivastigmine (Exelon), and galantamine (Razadyne) increase acetylcholine at cholinergic synapses by inhibiting its breakdown by acetylcholinesterase, which increases the availability of acetylcholine at neurotransmitter receptor sites in the CNS.

    - Therapeutic uses of these medications include the client's improved ability to perform self-care and slow cognitive deterioration of Alzheimer's disease for clients with mild to moderate Alzheimer's dementia.

SIDE/ADVERSE EFFECTS	NURSING INTERVENTIONS/CLIENT EDUCATION
Nausea and diarrhea, which occur in approximately 10% of clients	• Monitor for gastrointestinal side effects and for fluid volume deficits. • Promote adequate fluid intake. • The provider may titrate the dosage to reduce symptoms.
Bradycardia	• Teach the family to monitor pulse rate for the client who lives at home. • The client should be screened for underlying heart disease.

- Contraindications/precautions

  □ The cholinesterase inhibitors should be used with caution in clients with pre-existing asthma or other obstructive pulmonary disorders. Bronchoconstriction may be caused by an increase of acetylcholine.

MEDICATION/FOOD INTERACTIONS	NURSING INTERVENTIONS/CLIENT EDUCATION
Concurrent use of NSAIDs, such as aspirin, may cause gastrointestinal bleeding.	• Assess the use of over-the-counter NSAIDS. • Monitor for signs and symptoms of gastrointestinal bleeding.
Antihistamines, tricyclic antidepressants, and conventional antipsychotics (medications that block cholinergic receptors) can reduce the therapeutic effects of donepezil.	• Use of cholinergic receptor blocking medications for clients taking any cholinesterase inhibitor is not recommended.

- Nursing considerations
  - Dosage should start low and gradually be increased until side effects are no longer tolerable or medication is no longer beneficial.
  - Monitor for adverse effects and educate the client and family about these effects. Taper medication when discontinuing to prevent abrupt progression of symptoms.
  - Monitor the client for the ability to swallow tablets. Most of the medications are available in tablets and oral solutions. Donepezil is available in an orally disintegrating tablet.
  - Administer with or without food.
  - Donepezil has a long half-life and is administered once daily at bedtime. The other cholinesterase inhibitors are usually administered twice daily.

  o Medications, such as memantine (Namenda) block the entry of calcium into nerve cells, thus slowing down brain-cell death.

  - Memantine is the only medication approved for moderate to severe stages of Alzheimer's disease.
  - Nursing considerations
    - Memantine may be used concurrently with a cholinesterase inhibitor.
    - Administer the medication with or without food.
    - Monitor for common side effects, including dizziness, headache, confusion, and constipation.

- Alternative/Complementary Therapies
  - Estrogen therapy for women may prevent Alzheimer's disease, but it is not useful in decreasing the effects of pre-existing dementia.
  - Ginkgo biloba, an herbal product, is used by some clients memory. Instruct clients to inform the provider of the use of ginkgo biloba due to potential interactions, such as the risk for bleeding in clients taking antiplatelet medications, as well as the risk for seizures in clients taking medications that may lower seizure threshold.

- Care After Discharge
  - Educate family/caregivers about the client's illness, methods of care, and adaptation of the home environment.
  - Ensure a safe environment in the home. Questions to ask include:
    - Will the client wander out into the street if doors are left unlocked?
    - Is the client able to remember his address and his name?
    - Does the client harm others when allowed to wander in a long-term care facility?

- o Home safety measures to be implemented may include:
  - Removing scatter rugs
  - Installing door locks that cannot be easily opened
  - Locking water heater thermostat and turning water temperature down to a safe level
  - Providing good lighting, especially on stairs
  - Installing a handrail on stairs, and marking step edges with colored tape.
  - Placing mattresses on the floor
  - Removing clutter, keeping clear, wide pathways for walking through a room
  - Securing electrical cords to baseboards
  - Storing cleaning supplies in locked cupboards
  - Installing handrails in bathrooms
  - o Monitor for improvement in memory and the client's quality of life.

- Support for Caregivers
  - o Determine teaching needs for the client and especially the client's family members as the client's cognitive ability progressively declines.
  - o Review the resources available to the family as the client's health declines. Include long-term care options. A wide variety of home care and community resources may be available to the family in many areas of the country, and these resources may allow the client to remain at home, rather than in an institution.
  - o Provide support for caregivers. Recommend local support groups for caregivers, as well as respite care.
  - o Establish a routine. Make sure all caregivers know and apply the routine. Attempt to have consistency in caregivers.

- Client Outcomes
  - o The client will demonstrate improvement in cognition, memory, and ability to perform self-care.
  - o The client will remain free from injury.

CHAPTER 16: COGNITIVE DISORDERS

 Application Exercises

Scenario: An older adult client has just been diagnosed with stage 3 Alzheimer's disease. He is experiencing short-term memory loss, and his wife has quit her job to stay home with him because he is depressed and is also distressed about being so forgetful. The client just began taking donepezil (Aricept) 5 mg daily at bedtime.

1. How does donepezil (Aricept) work, and what are the benefits of the medication for this client?

2. The client's wife asks if donepezil will help treat her husband's depression, which she feels is worsening progressively as he becomes more forgetful. How should the nurse reply?

Scenario: An older adult client with stage 4 Alzheimer's disease lives with her husband, who is her primary caregiver. The client is often disoriented to time and place, and frequently talks about wanting to go someplace other than where she is. Her husband is fearful that she will wander outside or injure herself in the home.

3. When making a home visit, the nurse assesses the home for safety. Which of the following are appropriate suggestions to make to the client's husband to decrease the client's risk for injury?

4. During the home visit, the nurse determines that because the client's husband is the sole caregiver, he does not leave the house very often. Which of the following interventions should the nurse implement?

5. A client is admitted to an acute care facility with delirium caused by a severe urinary tract infection. Which of the following assessment data should the nurse expect to find? (Select all that apply.)

_____ No change in level of consciousness

_____ Perceptual disturbances

_____ Disorientation to time, place, person

_____ Stable vital signs

_____ Restlessness

CHAPTER 16: COGNITIVE DISORDERS

 Application Exercises Answer Key

Scenario: An older adult client has just been diagnosed with stage 3 Alzheimer's disease. He is experiencing short-term memory loss, and his wife has quit her job to stay home with him because he is depressed and is also distressed about being so forgetful. The client just began taking donepezil (Aricept) 5 mg daily at bedtime.

1. How does donepezil (Aricept) work, and what are the benefits of the medication for this client?

> **Cholinesterase inhibitors prevent the breakdown of acetylcholine in cerebral neurons, increasing its availability in the brain. Donepezil and the other cholinesterase inhibitors slow memory loss and improve behavior and daily function. Their use slows the progression of the disease for a few months and is effective in 30 to 60% of clients who take them.**

 NCLEX® Connection: Pharmacological and Parenteral Therapies, Expected Effects/Outcomes

2. The client's wife asks if donepezil will help treat her husband's depression, which she feels is worsening progressively as he becomes more forgetful. How should the nurse reply?

> **Cholinesterase inhibitors do not affect a client's mood. This client should be referred to his provider for possible placement on an antidepressant medication.**

 NCLEX® Connection: Pharmacological and Parenteral Therapies, Expected Effects/Outcomes

Scenario: An older adult client with stage 4 Alzheimer's disease lives with her husband, who is her primary caregiver. The client is often disoriented to time and place, and frequently talks about wanting to go someplace other than where she is. Her husband is fearful that she will wander outside or injure herself in the home.

3. When making a home visit, the nurse assesses the home for safety. Which of the following are appropriate suggestions to make to the client's husband to decrease the client's risk for injury?

> **Removing scatter rugs**
>
> **Installing door locks that cannot be easily opened**
>
> **Locking water heater thermostat and turning water temperature down to a safe level**
>
> **Providing good lighting, especially on stairs**
>
> **Installing a handrail on stairs, and marking step edges with colored tape**
>
> **Placing mattresses on the floor**
>
> **Removing clutter, keeping clear, wide pathways for walking through a room**
>
> **Securing electrical cords to baseboards**
>
> **Storing cleaning supplies in locked cupboards**
>
> **Installing handrails in bathrooms**

4. During the home visit, the nurse determines that because the client's husband is the sole caregiver, he does not leave the house very often. Which of the following interventions should the nurse implement?

Explore the possibility with the client's husband of asking relatives to provide respite care a few hours each week.

Encourage the caregiver to attend a local support group.

Obtain a referral for adult day care.

Provide information about long-term care options.

 NCLEX® Connection: Psychosocial Integrity, Mental Health Concepts

---

5. A client is admitted to an acute care facility with delirium caused by a severe urinary tract infection. Which of the following assessment data should the nurse expect to find? (Select all that apply)

	No change in level of consciousness
X	**Perceptual disturbances**
X	**Disorientation to time, place, person**
	Stable vital signs
X	**Restlessness**

The client with delirium may have perceptual disturbances, such as hallucinations and illusions; be disoriented to time, place, and person; and demonstrate restlessness. The client with delirium will likely have a change in level of consciousness and unstable vital signs, usually due to a medical condition.

 NCLEX® Connection: Psychosocial Integrity, Mental Health Concepts

UNIT 3	PSYCHOBIOLOGIC DISORDERS
Chapter 17	Chemical and Other Dependencies

Overview

- The various substance abuse and dependence disorders recognized and defined by the DSM-IV-TR include the following:

  - Substance abuse, which involves a repeated use of chemical substances, leading to clinically significant impairment over a 12-month period, and at least one of the following problems:

    - Inability to perform normal duties at home, school, and/or work.

    - Taking part in hazardous situations while impaired, such as driving.

    - Repeated legal or other personal problems caused by the substance use, such as losing one's job due to missed work time.

    - Continued use of the substance, despite the problems it has caused.

  - Substance dependence, which involves repeated use of chemical substances, leading to clinically significant impairment over a 12-month period, and three or more of the following:

    - The presence of tolerance – A need for higher and higher doses of a substance to achieve the desired effect, such as requiring larger amounts of alcohol to feel euphoric

    - The phenomenon of withdrawal – The stopping or reduction of intake that results in specific physical and psychological signs and symptoms, such as tremors, headaches, and other symptoms when the substance is not available

    - The substance taken in larger amounts or for longer periods than intended, such as continuing to take a prescribed opioid after surgical pain has ceased

    - A persistent (but unsuccessful) desire to control use of the substance

    - Progressively more time spent in obtaining, using, and recovering from use of the substance

    - Reduction in normal social or occupational activities

    - Continued use of the substance despite the problems it has caused

- Non-substance related dependency (process addictions), which dependence is on a behavior, examples

  - Gambling

  - Sexual behaviors

  - Shopping/spending

  - Internet use

- Addiction is characterized by:

  - Loss of control due to participation in the dependency, whether that dependency is on a substance or to a process

  - Participation in the dependency despite continuing associated problems

  - A tendency to relapse back into the dependency

- The defense mechanism of denial is commonly used by clients who have problems with drug abuse or dependency. For example, a person with long-term nicotine abuse might say, "I can quit whenever I want to, but smoking really doesn't cause me any problems." Frequently, denial prevents a client from obtaining help with substance or process abuse or dependency.

Assessment

- Risk Factors

  - Genetics – Predisposition to developing a dependency disorder due to family history

  - Lowered self-esteem

  - Lowered tolerance for pain and frustration

  - Few meaningful personal relationships

  - Few life successes

  - Risk-taking tendencies

  - Sociocultural theories

    - Certain cultures within the United States, such as Native American groups, have a high percentage of members with alcohol dependence. Other cultures, such as Asian groups, have a low percentage of alcohol dependence.

    - Peer pressure and other sociologic factors can increase the likelihood of substance use.

  - The older adult client may have a history of alcohol abuse or may develop a pattern of alcohol/substance abuse later in life due to life stressors, such as losing a spouse or a friend, retirement, or social isolation.

- Subjective and Objective Data

  o The nursing history should include the following:

    ▪ Type of substance or compulsive behavior

    ▪ Pattern and frequency of substance use

    ▪ Amount of substance used

    ▪ Age at onset of substance abuse

    ▪ Changes in use patterns

    ▪ Periods of abstinence in history

    ▪ Previous withdrawal symptoms

    ▪ Date of last substance use/compulsive behavior

    ▪ Review of systems:

      ☐ Blackout or loss of consciousness

      ☐ Changes in bowel movements

      ☐ Weight loss or weight gain

      ☐ Experience of stressful situation

      ☐ Sleep problems

      ☐ Chronic pain

      ☐ Concern over substance abuse

      ☐ Cutting down on consumption or behavior

  Ⓖ o The older adult client

    ▪ Alcohol use can lead to falls and other injuries, memory loss, somatic reports (headaches), and changes in sleep patterns.

    ▪ Alcohol dependence may include a decrease in ability for self-care (functional status), urinary incontinence, and signs of dementia.

    ▪ Older adults may show symptoms of alcohol abuse at lower doses than younger adults.

    ▪ Exposure to multiple medications in addition to age-related physiological changes raises the likelihood of adverse effects, such as confusion and falls.

- Central Nervous System Depressants
  - CNS depressants can produce physiological and psychological dependence and may have cross-tolerance, cross-dependency, and an additive effect when take concurrently.
    - Alcohol (ethanol)
      - A laboratory blood alcohol concentration (BAC) of 0.08% (80 g/dL) is considered legally intoxicated for adults operating automobiles in every U.S. state. Death could occur from acute toxicity in levels greater than about 0.35% (350 g/dL).
      - BAC depends on many factors, including body weight, gender, concentration of alcohol in drinks, number of drinks, gastric absorption rate, and the individual's tolerance level.

INTENDED EFFECTS	TOXIC EFFECTS	WITHDRAWAL SIGNS/SYMPTOMS
• Relaxation, decreased social anxiety, maintaining calm	• Effects of excess – altered judgment, decreased motor skills, decreased level of consciousness (which can include stupor or coma), respiratory arrest, peripheral collapse, and death (can occur with large doses) • Chronic use – direct cardiovascular damage, liver damage (ranging from fatty liver to cirrhosis), erosive gastritis and GI bleeding, acute pancreatitis, sexual dysfunction	• Effects usually start within 4 to 12 hr of the last intake of alcohol, peak after 24 to 48 hr, and then suddenly disappear. • Symptoms include abdominal cramping, vomiting, tremors, restlessness and inability to sleep, increased heart rate, blood pressure, respiratory rate, temperature, and tonic-clonic seizures. • Alcohol withdrawal delirium may occur 2 to 3 days after cessation of alcohol and may last 2 to 3 days. This is considered a medical emergency. Symptoms include severe disorientation, psychotic symptoms (hallucinations), severe hypertension, cardiac dysrhythmias, and delirium. Symptoms may progress to death.

- Benzodiazepines – Such as diazepam (Valium), can be taken orally or injected.

INTENDED EFFECTS	TOXIC EFFECTS	WITHDRAWAL SIGNS/SYMPTOMS
• Decreased anxiety, sedation	• Increased drowsiness and sedation, agitation, disorientation, nausea, vomiting • Respiratory depression • An antidote, flumazenil (Romazicon), available for IV use for benzodiazepine toxicity • Rapid dependence	• Anxiety, insomnia, diaphoresis, hypertension, possible psychotic reactions, and sometimes seizure activity

- Barbiturates – Such as pentobarbital (Nembutal) or secobarbital (Seconal) can be ingested orally and injected.

INTENDED EFFECTS	TOXIC EFFECTS	WITHDRAWAL SIGNS/SYMPTOMS
• Sedation, decreased anxiety	• Respiratory depression and decreased level of consciousness, which may be fatal • No antidote to reverse barbiturate toxicity	• Milder symptoms – The same as those seen in alcohol withdrawal • Severe symptoms – Possibly life-threatening convulsions, delirium, and cardiovascular collapse similar to that of alcohol withdrawal

- Cannabis – Marijuana or hashish (which is more potent), can be smoked or eaten

INTENDED EFFECTS	TOXIC EFFECTS	WITHDRAWAL SIGNS/SYMPTOMS
• Euphoria, sedation, hallucinations, decrease of nausea and vomiting secondary to chemotherapy, management of chronic pain	• Chronic use – Lung cancer, chronic bronchitis, and other respiratory effects • In high doses, occurrence of paranoia, such as delusions and hallucinations	• Possibly some depression

- Central Nervous System Stimulants
  - The CNS stimulation seen in specific CNS stimulants is dependent on the area of the brain and spinal cord affected.
    - Cocaine – Can be injected, smoked, or inhaled (snorted).

INTENDED EFFECTS	TOXIC EFFECTS	WITHDRAWAL SIGNS/SYMPTOMS
• Rush of euphoria and pleasure, increased energy	• Mild toxicity – Dizziness, irritability, tremor, blurred vision • Severe effects – Hallucinations, seizures, extreme fever, tachycardia, hypertension, chest pain, possible cardiovascular collapse and death	• Characteristic withdrawal syndrome occurring within 1 hr to several days of cessation of drug use • Depression, fatigue, craving, excess sleeping or insomnia, dramatic unpleasant dreams, psychomotor retardation or agitation • Not life threatening, but possible occurrence of suicidal ideation

- Amphetamines – Can be taken orally, injected intravenously, or smoked.

INTENDED EFFECTS	TOXIC EFFECTS	WITHDRAWAL SIGNS/SYMPTOMS
• Increased energy, euphoria similar to cocaine	• Impaired judgment, psychomotor agitation, hypervigilance, extreme irritability • Acute cardiovascular effects (tachycardia, elevated blood pressure), which could cause death	• Craving, depression, fatigue, sleeping (similar to those of cocaine) • Not life threatening

- Nicotine – Cigarettes and cigars are inhaled; smokeless tobacco is snuffed or chewed.

INTENDED EFFECTS	TOXIC EFFECTS	WITHDRAWAL SIGNS/SYMPTOMS
• Relaxation, decreased anxiety	• Highly toxic, but acute toxicity seen only in children or when exposure is to nicotine in pesticides • Also contains other harmful chemicals that are highly toxic and have long-term effects • Long-term effects: cardiovascular disease (hypertension, stroke) respiratory disease (emphysema, lung cancer); with smokeless tobacco (snuff or "chew"): irritation to oral mucous membranes and cancer	• Abstinence syndrome is evidenced by irritability, craving, nervousness, restlessness, anxiety, insomnia, increased appetite, and difficulty concentrating

- Opioids – Such as heroin, morphine, hydromorphone (Dilaudid) can be injected, smoked, and inhaled.

INTENDED EFFECTS	TOXIC EFFECTS	WITHDRAWAL SIGNS/SYMPTOMS
• A rush of euphoria (extreme well-being), relief from pain	• Decreased respirations and level of consciousness, which may cause death • An antidote, naloxone (Narcan), available for IV use to relieve symptoms of overdose	• Abstinence syndrome begins with sweating and rhinorrhea progressing to piloerection (gooseflesh), tremors, and irritability followed by severe weakness, nausea and vomiting, pain in the muscles and bones, and muscle spasms. • Withdrawal is very unpleasant but not life-threatening, and it is self-limiting to 7 to 10 days.

- Inhalants – Such as amyl nitrate, nitrous oxide, and solvents, are "sniffed," "huffed," or "bagged," often by young children or teenagers.

INTENDED EFFECTS	TOXIC EFFECTS	WITHDRAWAL SIGNS/SYMPTOMS
• Euphoria	• Depend on the drug, but generally can cause CNS depression, symptoms of psychosis (hallucinations), respiratory depression, and possible death	• None

- Hallucinogens – Such as lysergic acid diethylamide (LSD), mescaline (peyote), and phencyclidine piperidine (PCP) are usually ingested orally, can be injected or smoked.

INTENDED EFFECTS	TOXIC EFFECTS	WITHDRAWAL SIGNS/SYMPTOMS
• Heightened sense of self and altered perceptions (colors being more vivid while under the influence)	• Panic attacks, flashbacks (visual disturbances or hallucinations) which can occur intermittently for years	• None

- Illegal drugs continue to increase in potency, which increases the risk for onset of mental illness and major medical problems.

- Standardized Screening Tools

  o MAST (Michigan Alcohol Screening Test) or MAST-G (Michigan Alcohol Screening Test – Geriatric)

  o Addiction Severity Index

  o Recovery Attitude and Treatment Evaluator

  o Brief Drug Abuse Screen Test

  o CAGE-AID – This screening tool asks questions of the client to determine how the client perceives his current substance use.

Collaborative Care

- Nursing Care

  o The nurse must self-assess his own feelings regarding abuses, as those feelings may be transferred to the client through body language and the terminology the nurse may use in assessing the client. An objective, nonjudgmental approach by the nurse is imperative.

  o Use open-ended questions, such as "When was your last drink?"

- o Safety is the primary focus of nursing care during the acute stage of abuse.

  - Maintain a safe environment to prevent falls; implement seizure precautions as necessary.

  - Provide close observation for withdrawal symptoms, possibly one-on-one supervision. Physical restraint should be a last resort.

  - Orient the client to time, place, and person.

  - Maintain adequate nutrition and fluid balance.

  - Create a low-stimulation environment.

  - Administer withdrawal medications as prescribed.

  - Monitor for covert substance abuse during the detoxification period.

- o Provide emotional support and reassurance to the client and family.

  - Educate the client and family about codependent behaviors.

- o Begin to educate the client and family about addiction and the initial treatment goal of abstinence.

- o Educate the client and family regarding removing any prescription medications in the home that are not being used. And encourage the client not to share medication with someone for whom that medication is not prescribed.

- o Begin to develop motivation and commitment for abstinence and recovery (abstinence plus working a program of personal growth and self-discovery).

- o Encourage self-responsibility.

- o Help the client develop an emergency plan – a list of things the client would need to do and people he would need to contact.

- o Encourage attendance at self-help groups.

- Interdisciplinary Care

  - o Dual diagnosis, or comorbidity, means that an individual has both a mental illness, such as depression, as well as a problem with substance or process abuse. Both disorders need to be treated simultaneously and will require a team approach.

  - o Individual psychotherapies

    - Cognitive behavioral therapies, such as relaxation techniques or cognitive reframing, can be used to decrease anxiety and change behavior.

  - o Group therapy

    - Groups of clients with similar diagnoses may meet in an outpatient setting or within mental health residential facilities.

- o Family therapy
    - This therapy identifies codependency, which is a common behavior demonstrated by the significant other/family/friends of an individual with substance or process dependency, and assists the family to change that behavior. The codependent person reacts in overresponsible ways that actually allow the dependent individual to continue the substance (or process) abuse or dependency. For example, a spouse may call the client's employer with an excuse of illness when the client is actually intoxicated
    - Families learn about abuse of specific substances.
    - The client and family are educated regarding such issues as family coping, problem solving, relapse signs, and availability of support groups.
- Pharmacological therapy
    - o Medications
        - Alcohol withdrawal – Diazepam (Valium), lorazepam (Ativan), carbamazepine (Tegretol), clonidine (Catapres)
        - Alcohol abstinence – Disulfiram (Antabuse), naltrexone (Revia), acamprosate (Campral)
        - Opioid withdrawal – methadone (Dolophine) substitution, clonidine (Catapres), buprenorphine (Subutex), buprenorphine combined with naloxone Suboxone)
        - Nicotine withdrawal – Bupropion (Zyban), nicotine replacement therapy (nicotine gum [Nicorette] and nicotine patch [Nicotrol])
        - Nursing Considerations
            - □ Monitor the client's vital signs and neurological status.
            - □ Provide for client safety by implementing seizure precautions
        - Client Education
            - □ Encourage the client to adhere to the treatment plan
            - □ Advise client taking disulfiram to avoid all alcohol
- Care After Discharge
    - o Client Education
        - Teach the client to recognize signs/symptoms of relapse and factors that contribute to relapse.
        - Teach cognitive-behavioral techniques to help maintain sobriety and to create feelings of pleasure from activities other than using substances, or from process addictions.
        - Assist the client to develop communication skills to communicate with coworkers and family members while sober.

- Encourage the client and family to attend a 12-step program, such as Alcoholics Anonymous (AA), Narcotics Anonymous, Gambler's Anonymous, and family groups like Al-Anon or Ala-Teen.

  - These programs will teach clients the following:

    - Abstinence is necessary for recovery.

    - A higher power is needed to assist in recovery.

    - They are not responsible for their disease but are responsible for their recovery.

    - Others cannot be blamed for their addictions and they must acknowledge their feelings and problems.

- Client Outcomes

  - The client will verbalize coping strategies to use in times of stress.

  - The client will remain substance free.

  - The client will remain free from injury.

  - The client will attend a 12-step program regularly.

CHAPTER 17: CHEMICAL AND OTHER DEPENDENCIES

(A) Application Exercises

Scenario: A 45-year-old client was admitted to an acute care facility for medically supervised detoxification 8 hr ago. The client was admitted because he was involved in a motor vehicle crash while driving under the influence of alcohol. Assessment findings reveal no physical injury, a blood alcohol concentration (BAC) of 200 g/dL (0.20%), and a 30-year history of alcohol abuse. He has been in rehabilitation facilities several times but has always relapsed. He lives alone after a separation from his wife and three teenage children, whom the client has not seen in a year. The client has not been able to keep a job due to poor attendance, and he has been out of work for the past 6 months. The client also has additional driving-under-the-influence (DUI) citations.

1. According to the DSM-IV-TR, what signs of substance dependence does this client have?

2. When assessing the client for alcohol withdrawal, which of the following observations should the nurse expect to make? (Select all that apply.)

    _____   Bradycardia

    _____   Fine tremors of both hands

    _____   Hypotension

    _____   Vomiting

    _____   Restlessness

3. Which of the following interventions is the highest priority for the client at this time?

    A. Orient the client to time, place, and person as needed.

    B. Offer fluids and nourishing diet as tolerated.

    C. Implement seizure precautions.

    D. Encourage participation in group therapy sessions.

4. Which of the following medications should the nurse anticipate administering to assist the client with maintaining abstinence from alcohol?

    A. Chlordiazepoxide (Librium)

    B. Bupropion (Zyban)

    C. Disulfiram (Antabuse)

    D. Carbamazepine (Tegretol)

CHAPTER 17: CHEMICAL AND OTHER DEPENDENCIES

(A) Application Exercises Answer Key

Scenario: A 45-year-old client was admitted to an acute care facility for medically supervised detoxification 8 hr ago. The client was admitted because he was involved in a motor vehicle crash while driving under the influence of alcohol. Assessment findings reveal no physical injury, a blood alcohol concentration (BAC) of 200 g/dL (0.20%), and a 30-year history of alcohol abuse. He has been in rehabilitation facilities several times but has always relapsed. He lives alone after a separation from his wife and three teenage children, whom the client has not seen in a year. The client has not been able to keep a job due to poor attendance, and he has been out of work for the past 6 months. The client also has additional driving-under-the-influence (DUI) citations.

1. According to the DSM-IV-TR, what signs of substance dependence does this client have?

Several attempts to stop drinking unsuccessful
Reduction in normal social or occupational activities – estranged from family and unable to work
Continued use of the substance despite the problems it has caused

(N) NCLEX® Connection: Psychosocial Integrity: Chemical and Other Dependencies

2. When assessing the client for alcohol withdrawal, which of the following observations should the nurse expect to make? (Select all that apply.)

	Bradycardia
X	**Fine tremors of both hands**
	Hypotension
X	**Vomiting**
X	**Restlessness**

Tremors ,vomiting, restlessness and inability to sleep, depressed mood, and/or irritability are all expected findings for a client who is experiencing alcohol withdrawal. Vital signs are usually increased, and therefore, the client will most likely have tachycardia and elevated blood pressure.

(N) NCLEX® Connection: Psychosocial Integrity: Chemical and Other Dependencies

3. Which of the following interventions is the highest priority for the client at this time?

    A. Orient the client to time, place, and person as needed.

    B. Offer fluids and nourishing diet as tolerated.

    C. Implement seizure precautions.

    D. Encourage participation in group therapy sessions.

The greatest risk to the client at this time is injury from seizures and falls. Therefore, implementing seizure precautions is the highest priority to prevent injury in case of occurrence of a seizure. Keeping the client oriented, offering fluids and a nourishing diet, and encouraging participation in group therapy sessions are all important but are not the highest priority at this time.

Ⓝ NCLEX® Connection: Safety and Infection Control: Injury Prevention

4. Which of the following medications should the nurse anticipate administering to assist the client with maintaining abstinence from alcohol?

    A. Chlordiazepoxide (Librium)

    B. Bupropion (Zyban)

    C. Disulfiram (Antabuse)

    D. Carbamazepine (Tegretol)

Disulfiram is administered to help the client maintain abstinence from alcohol. If the client drinks alcohol while taking disulfiram, she may experience a mild reaction, such as nausea and vomiting, or a more severe reaction that can lead to respiratory depression and death. Chlordiazepoxide and carbamazepine are administered for acute alcohol withdrawal. Bupropion is administered for nicotine withdrawal.

Ⓝ NCLEX® Connection: Pharmacological and Parenteral Therapies: Expected Effects/Outcomes

UNIT 3   PSYCHOBIOLOGIC DISORDERS

Chapter 18   Eating Disorders

Overview

- The various eating disorders recognized and defined by the DSM-IV-TR include the following:

  o   Anorexia nervosa

    ■   Clients are preoccupied with food and the rituals of eating, along with a voluntary refusal to eat.

    ■   Clients exhibit a morbid fear of obesity and a refusal to maintain a minimally normal body weight (Body weight is less than 85% of expected normal weight for the individual.) in the absence of a physical cause.

    ■   This condition occurs most often in females from adolescence to young adulthood. Only 5% to 10% of clients who have anorexia nervosa are male.

    ■   Two types:

      □   Restricting type – The individual drastically restricts food intake and does not binge or purge.

      □   Binge-eating/purging type – The individual engages in binge eating or purging behaviors.

  o   Bulimia nervosa

    ■   Clients recurrently eat large quantities of food over a short period of time (bingeing), which may be followed by inappropriate compensatory behaviors, such as self-induced vomiting (purging), to rid the body of the excess calories.

    ■   Most clients with bulimia maintain a weight within a normal range or slightly higher.

    ■   The average age of onset in females is 15 to 18 years of age.

    ■   About 10% to 15% of clients with bulimia are males. Onset generally occurs between 18 and 26 years of age, and bingeing with the use of excessive exercise (nonpurging type) is most common.

    ■   Two types:

      □   Purging type, in which the client uses self-induced vomiting, laxatives, diuretics, and/or enemas to lose or maintain weight

      □   Nonpurging type, in which the client may also compensate for bingeing through other means, such as excessive exercise and the misuse of laxatives, diuretics, and/or enemas

- Mortality rate for eating disorders is high and suicide is also a risk.

- Treatment modalities focus on normalizing eating patterns and beginning to address the issues raised by the illness.

- Comorbidities include major depressive disorder and dysthymia (50% - 75%), obsessive compulsive disorder, substance abuse, and anxiety disorders.

Assessment

- Risk Factors
  - Females
    - Family genetics – more commonly seen in families with sisters and mothers with eating disorders
    - Biological – hypothalamic, neurotransmitter, hormonal, or biochemical imbalance, with disturbances of the serotonin neurotransmitter pathways seeming to be implicated
    - Interpersonal relationships – influenced by parental pressure and the need to succeed
    - Psychological influences – rigidity, ritualism; separation and individuation conflicts; feelings of ineffectiveness, helplessness, and depression; and distorted body image
    - Environmental factors – pressure from society to have the "perfect body," culture of abundance
    - Individual history of being a "picky" eater in childhood
    - Participation in athletics, especially at an elite level of competition
  - Males
    - Participation in a sport where lean body build is prized (bicycling) or where a specific weight is necessary (wrestling)
    - A history of obesity
- Subjective and Objective Data
  - Nursing history should include the following:
    - The client's perception of the issue
    - Eating habits
    - History of dieting
    - Methods of weight control (restricting, purging, exercising)
    - Value attached to a specific shape and weight
    - Interpersonal and social functioning
    - Difficulty with impulsivity, as well as compulsivity

■ Family and interpersonal relationships (frequently troublesome and chaotic, reflecting a lack of nurturing)

OBJECTIVE DATA	FINDINGS
Mental status	• Cognitive distortions include: 　○ Overgeneralizations – "Other girls don't like me because I'm fat." 　○ "All-or-nothing" thinking – "If I eat any dessert, I'll gain 50 pounds." 　○ Catastrophizing – "My life is over if I gain weight." 　○ Personalization – "When I walk through the hospital hallway, I know everyone is looking at me." 　○ Emotional reasoning – "I know I look bad because I feel bloated." • Client demonstrates high interest in preparing food, but not eating. • Client is terrified of gaining weight. • Client perception is that she is severely overweight and sees this image reflected in the mirror. • Client may exhibit low self-esteem, impulsivity, difficulty with interpersonal relationships. • Client may participate in an intense physical regimen.
Vital signs	• Low blood pressure with possible orthostatic hypotension • Decreased pulse and body temperature
Weight	• Clients with anorexia have a body weight that is less than 85% of expected normal weight. • Most clients with bulimia maintain a weight within the normal range or slightly higher.
Skin, hair, and nails	Clients with anorexia may have fine, downy hair (lanugo) on the face and back; yellowed skin; mottled, cool extremities; and poor skin turgor.
Head, neck, mouth, and throat	• Enlargement of the parotid glands • Dental erosion and caries (if the client is purging)
Cardiovascular system	• Irregular heart rate (dysrhythmias noted on cardiac monitor), heart failure, cardiomyopathy • Peripheral edema
Musculoskeletal system	• Muscle weakness
Gastrointestinal system	• Constipation • Self-induced vomiting • Excessive use of diuretics or laxatives
Reproductive status	Anorexia is accompanied by amenorrhea for at least three consecutive cycles.

- o Criteria for inpatient treatment includes:
  - Rapid weight loss or weight loss of greater than 30% of body weight over 6 months
  - Unsuccessful weight gain in outpatient treatment, failure to adhere to treatment contract
  - Vital signs demonstrating heart rate less than 40 bpm, systolic blood pressure less than 70 mm Hg, body temperature less than 36° C (96.8° F)
  - ECG changes
  - Electrolyte disturbances
  - Severe depression
  - Suicidal behavior
  - Family crisis
- o Laboratory and diagnostic tests
  - Common laboratory abnormalities associated with anorexia include:
    - □ Hypokalemia, especially for those who are also bulimic
      - ‣ There is a direct loss of potassium due to purging (vomiting).
      - ‣ Dehydration stimulates increased aldosterone production, which leads to sodium and water retention and potassium excretion.
    - □ Anemia and leukopenia with lymphocytosis
    - □ Possible impaired liver function, shown by increased enzyme levels
    - □ Possible elevated cholesterol
    - □ Abnormal thyroid function tests
    - □ Elevated carotene levels, which cause skin to appear yellow
    - □ Decreased bone density (possible osteoporosis)
    - □ Abnormal blood glucose level
    - □ ECG changes
  - Electrolyte imbalances associated with bulimia are common and may depend on the client's method of purging (laxatives, diuretics, vomiting). Laboratory abnormalities include:
    - □ Hypokalemia
    - □ Hyponatremia
    - □ Hypochloremia
- o Standardized screening tools
  - Eating Disorders Inventory
  - Body Attitude Test
  - Diagnostic Survey for Eating Disorders

Collaborative Care

- Nursing Care

  - Provide a highly structured milieu in an inpatient eating disorder unit for the client requiring intensive therapy.

  - Develop and maintain a trusting nurse/client relationship through consistency and therapeutic communication.

  - Use a positive approach and support to promote client self-esteem and positive self-image.

  - Encourage client decision making and participation in the plan of care to allow for a sense of control.

  - Establish realistic goals for weight gain.

  - Promote cognitive-behavioral therapies:

    - Cognitive reframing

    - Relaxation techniques

    - Journal writing

    - Desensitization exercises

  - Monitor the client's vital signs, intake and output, and weight.

  - Use behavioral contracts to modify client behaviors.

  - Reward the client for positive behaviors, such as completing meals or consuming a set number of calories.

  - Closely monitor the client during and after meals to prevent purging, which may necessitate accompanying the client to the bathroom.

  - Monitor the client for maintenance of appropriate exercise.

  - Teach and encourage self-care activities.

  - Provide nutrition education to include correcting misinformation regarding food, meal planning, and food selection.

    - Consider the client's preferences and ability to consume food when developing the initial eating plan.

    - Establish a structured and inflexible eating schedule at the start of therapy, only permitting food during scheduled times.

    - Provide small, frequent meals, which are better tolerated and will help prevent the client from feeling overwhelmed.

    - Provide a diet high in fiber to control constipation.

    - Provide a diet low in sodium to control fluid retention.

    - Limit high-fat and gassy foods during the start of treatment.

- ■ Administer a multivitamin and mineral supplement.

- ■ Instruct the client to avoid caffeine.

- ○ Make arrangements for the client to attend individual, group, and family therapy to assist in resolving personal issues contributing to the eating disorder.

- Medications

  - ○ Selective serotonin reuptake inhibitors (SSRIs), such as fluoxetine (Prozac)

    - ■ Nursing Considerations

      - □ Instruct the client that medication may take 1 to 3 weeks for initial response, with up to 2 months for maximal response.

      - □ Instruct the client to avoid hazardous activities (driving, operating heavy equipment/machinery) until individual side effects are known.

      - □ Instruct the client to notify the provider if sexual dysfunction occurs and is intolerable.

- Interdisciplinary Care

  - ○ A registered dietitian should be involved to provide the client with nutritional and dietary guidance.

- Care After Discharge

  - ○ Assist the client to develop and implement a maintenance plan.

  - ○ Encourage follow-up treatment in an outpatient setting.

  - ○ Encourage client participation in a support group.

  - ○ Continue individual and family therapy as indicated.

- Client Outcomes

  - ○ The client will maintain agreed-upon weight goals.

  - ○ The client will establish normal eating habits.

  - ○ The client will verbalize a positive body image.

- Complications

  - ○ Refeeding syndrome

    - ■ Refeeding syndrome is the circulatory collapse that occurs when a client's completely compromised cardiac system is overwhelmed by a replenished vascular system after normal fluid intake resumes.

    - ■ Nursing actions:

      - □ Care for the client in a hospital setting.

      - □ Implement refeeding over at least 7 days.

      - □ Monitor serum electrolytes, and administer fluid replacement as prescribed.

- ○ Cardiac dysrhythmias, severe bradycardia, and hypotension
  - ▪ Nursing actions:
    - ☐ Place the client on continuous cardiac monitoring.
    - ☐ Monitor the client's vital signs frequently.
    - ☐ Report changes in the client's status to the provider.

CHAPTER 18: EATING DISORDERS

 Application Exercises

Scenario: A nurse is working with a 16-year-old client in a community mental health facility. The client and her mother have begun exploring colleges extensively. After school, the client spends her time preparing gourmet meals for her family while her mother is working. Lately, her mother has noticed that the client is not eating the food she prepares. Instead, she busies herself serving the rest of the family and says she is dieting in order to "have friends at college." During a recent physical examination, it was discovered that the client's weight dropped from an ideal weight for her height, 115 lb, to 95 lb in the past 3 months. She has also stopped menstruating. Her primary care provider has referred her to the mental health center for counseling.

1. What assessments are important for this client?

2. What physical symptoms of anorexia nervosa does this client have, and what other signs of the disorder does she display?

3. A client is hospitalized on an eating disorders unit. She has a history and current diagnosis of bulimia nervosa. Which of the following should the nurse expect to find? (Select all that apply.)

    _____ Hyperkalemia

    _____ Amenorrhea

    _____ ECG changes

    _____ Cool extremities

    _____ Peripheral edema

    _____ Yellowed skin

    _____ Weight within normal range or slightly higher

    _____ Hyponatremia

4. A client being treated for bulimia has stopped purging. She tells the nurse that she is afraid she is going to gain weight. Which of the following is an appropriate response by the nurse?

    A. "You don't need to be concerned. The dietitian will ensure that you don't get too many calories in your diet."

    B. "Don't worry about your weight. We are going to work on other problems while you are in the hospital."

    C. "I understand you have concerns about your weight, but right now I want you to tell me about your recent invitation to join the National Honor Society. That's quite an accomplishment."

    D. "You are not overweight, and the staff will ensure that you do not gain weight while you are in the hospital. We know that is important to you."

CHAPTER 18: EATING DISORDERS

 Application Exercises Answer Key

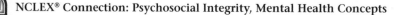

Scenario: A nurse is working with a 16-year-old client in a community mental health facility. The client and her mother have begun exploring colleges extensively. After school, the client spends her time preparing gourmet meals for her family while her mother is working. Lately, her mother has noticed that the client is not eating the food she prepares. Instead, she busies herself serving the rest of the family and says she is dieting in order to "have friends at college." During a recent physical examination, it was discovered that the client's weight dropped from an ideal weight for her height, 115 lb, to 95 lb in the past 3 months. She has also stopped menstruating. Her primary care provider has referred her to the mental health center for counseling.

1. What assessments are important for this client?

Dietary habits and history

Height and weight

Condition of skin

Physical assessment parameters, such as vital signs

Feelings about body image

Family dynamics

 NCLEX® Connection: Psychosocial Integrity, Mental Health Concepts

2. What physical symptoms of anorexia nervosa does this client have, and what other signs of the disorder does she display?

This client has weight loss greater than 15% of her ideal body weight, and she has amenorrhea. She also is interested in food (cooks for the family and serves the food) but does not eat it. From the data in the scenario, it appears this client has anorexia nervosa, nonpurging type.

 NCLEX® Connection: Psychosocial Integrity, Mental Health Concepts

3. A client is hospitalized on an eating disorders unit. She has a history of and current diagnosis of bulimia nervosa. Which of the following should the nurse expect to find? (Select all that apply.)

_____	Hyperkalemia
_____	Amenorrhea
X	**ECG changes**
_____	Cool extremities
X	**Peripheral edema**
_____	Yellowed skin
X	**Weight within normal range or slightly higher**
X	**Hyponatremia**

ECG changes, peripheral edema, weight within the normal range or slightly higher, and hyponatremia are all findings consistent with bulimia nervosa. The client with bulimia is more likely to have hypokalemia. Amenorrhea, cool extremities, and yellowed skin are findings consistent with anorexia nervosa.

(N) NCLEX® Connection: Psychosocial Integrity, Mental Health Concepts

4. A client being treated for bulimia has stopped purging. She tells the nurse that she is afraid she is going to gain weight. Which of the following is an appropriate response by the nurse?

A. "You don't need to be concerned. The dietitian will ensure that you don't get too many calories in your diet."

B. "Don't worry about your weight. We are going to work on other problems while you are in the hospital."

C. **"I understand you have concerns about your weight, but right now I want you to tell me about your recent invitation to join the National Honor Society. That's quite an accomplishment."**

D. "You are not overweight, and the staff will ensure that you do not gain weight while you are in the hospital. We know that is important to you."

In the correct option, the nurse acknowledges the client's concerns and then focuses the conversation on the client's accomplishment. The other options minimize the client's concerns about being overweight and/or gaining weight.

(N) NCLEX® Connection: Psychosocial Integrity, Behavioral Interventions

UNIT 4: PSYCHOPHARMACOLOGICAL THERAPIES

- Medications for Anxiety Disorders
- Medications for Depression
- Medications for Bipolar Disorders
- Medications for Psychoses
- Medications for Children and Adolescents With Mental Health Issues
- Medications for Substance Abuse

NCLEX® CONNECTIONS

When reviewing the chapters in this unit, keep in mind the relevant sections of the NCLEX® outline, in particular:

CLIENT NEEDS: PHARMACOLOGICAL AND PARENTERAL THERAPIES

Relevant topics/tasks include:
- Adverse Effects/Contraindications/Side Effects/Interactions
  - Monitor for anticipated interactions among the client prescribed medications and fluids.
- Expected Actions/Outcomes
  - Use clinical decision making/critical thinking when addressing expected effects/outcomes of medications.
- Medication Administration
  - Educate the client about medications.

UNIT 4	PSYCHOPHARMACOLOGICAL THERAPIES
Chapter 19	Medications for Anxiety Disorders

Overview

- The major medications used to treat anxiety disorders include:

  o Benzodiazepine sedative hypnotic anxiolytics, such as diazepam (Valium)

  o Atypical anxiolytic/nonbarbiturate anxiolytics, such as buspirone (BuSpar)

  o Selective serotonin reuptake inhibitors (SSRIs), such as paroxetine (Paxil)

- Other classifications that may be used include:

  o Antidepressants

    ▪ Amitriptyline (Elavil), a tricyclic antidepressant (TCA)

    ▪ Phenelzine (Nardil), a monoamine oxidase inhibitor (MAOI)

    ▪ Venlafaxine (Effexor), a serotonin-norepinephrine reuptake inhibitor (SSRI)

  o CNS stimulants, such as methylphenidate (Ritalin, Concerta)

  o Antihistamines, such as hydroxyzine pamoate (Vistaril)

  o Beta blockers, such as propranolol (Inderal)

  o Anticonvulsants, such as gabapentin (Neurontin)

MEDICATION CLASSIFICATION: BENZODIAZEPINE SEDATIVE HYPNOTIC ANXIOLYTICS

- Select Prototype Medication: Diazepam (Valium)

- Other Medications:

  o Alprazolam (Xanax)

  o Lorazepam (Ativan)

  o Chlordiazepoxide (Librium)

  o Clorazepate (Tranxene)

  o Oxazepam (Serax)

  o Clonazepam (Klonopin)

Purpose

- Expected Pharmacological Action

  o Diazepam enhances the inhibitory effects of gamma-aminobutyric acid (GABA) in the central nervous system. Relief from anxiety occurs rapidly following administration.

- Therapeutic Uses

  o Generalized anxiety disorder and panic disorder

  o Other uses for benzodiazepines include:

    ▪ Seizure disorders

    ▪ Insomnia

    ▪ Muscle spasm

    ▪ Alcohol withdrawal (for prevention and treatment of acute symptoms)

    ▪ Induction of anesthesia

Complications

SIDE/ADVERSE EFFECTS	NURSING INTERVENTIONS/CLIENT EDUCATION
CNS depression, such as sedation, light-headedness, ataxia, and decreased cognitive function	• Advise the client to observe for symptoms. Instruct the client to notify the provider if symptoms occur. • Advise the client to avoid hazardous activities (driving, operating heavy equipment/machinery).
Anterograde amnesia – difficulty recalling events that occur after dosing	• Advise the client to observe for symptoms. Instruct the client to notify the provider and stop the medication if symptoms occur.
Acute toxicity • Oral toxicity – drowsiness, lethargy, confusion • IV toxicity – respiratory depression, severe hypotension, cardiac arrest	• Advise the client to watch for manifestations of overdose. Notify the provider if these occur. • For oral toxicity, gastric lavage can be used, followed by the administration of activated charcoal or saline cathartics. • Flumazenil (Romazicon) can be administered to counteract sedation and reverse the side effects. • Monitor the client's vital signs, maintain patent airway, and provide fluids to maintain blood pressure. • Ensure availability of resuscitation equipment.

SIDE/ADVERSE EFFECTS	NURSING INTERVENTIONS/CLIENT EDUCATION
Paradoxical response (insomnia, excitation, euphoria, anxiety, rage)	• Advise the client to observe for symptoms. Instruct the client to notify the provider if symptoms occur.
Withdrawal symptoms, which occur infrequently with short-term use, such as anxiety, insomnia, diaphoresis, tremors, and light-headedness	• Advise the client who has been taking diazepam regularly and in high doses to taper the dose over several weeks.

Ⓢ Contraindications/Precautions

- Diazepam is a pregnancy risk category D medication.

- Benzodiazepines are classified under Schedule IV of the Controlled Substances Act.

- Diazepam is contraindicated in clients with sleep apnea and/or respiratory depression.

- Use diazepam cautiously in clients who have liver disease and/or a history of substance abuse.

Medication/Food Interactions

MEDICATION/FOOD INTERACTIONS	NURSING INTERVENTIONS/CLIENT EDUCATION
• CNS depressants, such as alcohol, barbiturates, and opioids may cause respiratory depression.	• Advise the client to observe for symptoms. Instruct the client to notify the provider if symptoms occur. • Advise the client to avoid hazardous activities (driving, operating heavy equipment/machinery).

Nursing Administration

- Advise the client to take the medication as prescribed, and to avoid abrupt discontinuation of treatment to prevent withdrawal symptoms.

- When discontinuing benzodiazepines that have been taken regularly for long periods and in higher doses, taper the dose over several weeks.

- Administer the medication with meals or snacks if GI upset occurs.

- Advise the client to swallow sustained-release tablets and to avoid chewing or crushing the tablets.

- Instruct the client about the potential for dependency during and after treatment and to notify the provider if symptoms occur.

MEDICATION CLASSIFICATION: ATYPICAL ANXIOLYTIC/NONBARBITURATE ANXIOLYTICS

- Select Prototype Medication: Buspirone (BuSpar)

Purpose

- Expected Pharmacological Action

  o The exact antianxiety mechanism of this medication is unknown. This medication does bind to serotonin and dopamine receptors. There is less potential for abuse than with other anxiolytics, and use of buspirone does not result in sedation or potentiate the effects of other CNS depressants.

- Therapeutic Uses

  o Panic disorder

  o Obsessive compulsive disorder

  o Social anxiety disorder

  o Posttraumatic stress disorder

Complications

SIDE/ADVERSE EFFECTS	NURSING INTERVENTIONS/CLIENT EDUCATION
CNS effects such as dizziness, nausea, headache, light-headedness, agitation	This medication does not interfere with activities, because it does not cause sedation.

Ⓢ Contraindications/Precautions

- Buspirone is a pregnancy risk category B medication.

- Buspirone is not recommended for use by nursing mothers.

- Use buspirone cautiously in older adult clients, as well as clients with liver and/or renal dysfunction.

- Buspirone is contraindicated for concurrent use with MAOI antidepressants, or for 14 days after MAOIs are discontinued. Hypertensive crisis may result.

Medication/Food interactions

MEDICATION/FOOD INTERACTIONS	NURSING INTERVENTIONS/CLIENT EDUCATION
Erythromycin, ketoconazole, and grapefruit juice may increase the effects of buspirone.	- Advise the client to avoid the use of erythromycin and ketoconazole. - Advise the client to avoid drinking grapefruit juice.

Nursing Administration

- Advise the client to take the medication with meals to prevent gastric irritation.

- Advise the client that effects do not occur immediately. It may take a week to notice first therapeutic effects, and several more weeks to reach full therapeutic benefit. Medication should be taken on a regular basis, rather than an as-needed basis.

- Instruct clients that tolerance, dependence, or withdrawal symptoms are not an issue with this medication.

MEDICATION CLASSIFICATION: SELECTIVE SEROTONIN REUPTAKE INHIBITORS (SSRIs)

- Select Prototype Medication: Paroxetine (Paxil)

- Other Medications:

  o Sertraline (Zoloft)

  o Escitalopram (Lexapro)

  o Fluoxetine (Prozac)

  o Fluvoxamine (Luvox)

  o Duloxetine (Cymbalta)

Purpose

- Expected Pharmacological Action

  o Paroxetine selectively inhibits serotonin reuptake, allowing more serotonin to stay at the junction of the neurons.

  o It does not block uptake of dopamine or norepinephrine.

  o Paroxetine causes CNS stimulation, which can cause insomnia.

  o The medication has a long effective half-life; about 4 weeks are necessary to produce therapeutic medication levels.

- Therapeutic Uses

  o Paroxetine

    ▪ Generalized anxiety disorder (GAD)

    ▪ Panic disorder – decreases both the frequency and intensity of panic attacks, and also prevents anticipatory anxiety about attacks

    ▪ Obsessive compulsive disorder (OCD) – reduces symptoms by increasing serotonin

    ▪ Social anxiety disorder

    ▪ Posttraumatic stress disorder

    ▪ Depressive disorders

- ○ Sertraline is indicated for panic disorder, OCD, social anxiety disorder, and PTSD.

- ○ Escitalopram is indicated for GAD and OCD.

- ○ Fluoxetine is used for panic disorder and GAD.

- ○ Fluvoxamine is used for OCD and social anxiety disorder.

- ○ Duloxetine is used for GAD.

Complications

SIDE/ADVERSE EFFECTS	NURSING INTERVENTIONS/CLIENT EDUCATION
Early adverse effects (first few days/weeks): nausea, diaphoresis, tremor, fatigue, drowsiness	• Advise the client that these effects should soon subside. • Instruct the client to report symptoms to the provider. • Instruct the client to take the medication as prescribed.
Later adverse effects (after 5 to 6 weeks of therapy): sexual dysfunction (e.g., impotence, delayed or absent orgasm, delayed or absent ejaculation, decreased sexual interest), weight gain, headache	• Instruct the client to report problems with sexual function (may be managed with dose reduction, medication holiday, changing medications).
Weight gain	• Advise the client to follow a well-balanced diet and exercise regularly.
Gastrointestinal bleeding	• Use cautiously in clients with a history of gastrointestinal bleed, ulcers, and those taking other medications that affect blood coagulation. • Advise the client to report signs of bleeding, such as dark stools, emesis that has the appearance of coffee grounds.
Hyponatremia – more likely in older adult clients taking diuretics	• Obtain baseline serum sodium, and monitor level periodically throughout treatment.
Serotonin syndrome • Agitation, confusion, disorientation, difficulty concentrating, anxiety, hallucinations, hyperreflexia, fever, diaphoresis, incoordination, tremors • Usually begins 2 to 72 hr after initiation of treatment • Resolves when the medication is discontinued	• Watch for and advise the client to report any of these symptoms, which could indicate a lethal problem.

SIDE/ADVERSE EFFECTS	NURSING INTERVENTIONS/CLIENT EDUCATION

Bruxism: grinding and clenching of teeth, usually during sleep	• Bruxism should be reported to the provider, who may:
	   ○ Switch the client to another class of medication.
	   ○ Treat bruxism with low-dose buspirone.
	   ○ Advise the client to use a mouth guard during sleep.

Withdrawal syndrome • Nausea, sensory disturbances, anxiety, tremor, malaise, unease • Minimized by tapering the medication slowly	• Advise the client that, after a long period of use, the medication will be tapered slowly to avoid withdrawal symptoms. • Advise the client to avoid abrupt discontinuation of the medication.

 Contraindications/Precautions

- Paroxetine is a pregnancy risk category D medication. Other SSRIs pose less risk during pregnancy.

- Paroxetine is contraindicated in clients taking MAOIs.

- Clients taking paroxetine should avoid alcohol.

- Use paroxetine cautiously in clients with liver and renal dysfunction, seizure disorders, or a history of gastrointestinal bleeding.

- Use SSRIs cautiously in clients who have bipolar disorder, due to the risk for mania.

Medication/Food Interactions

MEDICATION/FOOD INTERACTIONS	NURSING INTERVENTIONS/CLIENT EDUCATION
Concurrent use of MAOIs or tricyclic antidepressants with paroxetine can cause serotonin syndrome.	Advise the client to avoid concurrent use of these medications.

Nursing Administration

- Advise the client that paroxetine may be taken with food. Sleep disturbances may be minimized by taking the medication in the morning.

- Instruct the client to take the medication on a daily basis to establish therapeutic plasma levels.

- Assist the client with medication regimen adherence by informing the client that therapeutic effects may not be experienced for 1 to 3 weeks.

Nursing Evaluation of Medication Effectiveness

- Depending on therapeutic intent, effectiveness may be evidenced by:
    ○ Maintenance of a normal sleep pattern
    ○ Verbalization of feeling less anxious and more relaxed
    ○ Greater ability to participate in social and occupational interactions

CHAPTER 19: MEDICATIONS FOR ANXIETY DISORDERS

 Application Exercises

1. A nurse working in a mental health clinic is providing teaching to a client with a new prescription for diazepam (Valium) for generalized anxiety disorder. The client had originally told her provider that she took no other medications. However, before leaving the clinic, she says to the nurse, "Oh, I forgot that I do take a sleeping pill at night for insomnia, and I also usually drink a glass of wine before bedtime to make sure I sleep." What should be the nurse's concerns about this information, and what interventions are necessary?

2. Which of the following is an antidote for benzodiazepine overdose or toxicity?

   A. Buspirone (BuSpar)

   B. Venlafaxine (Effexor)

   C. Flumazenil (Romazicon)

   D. Naloxone (Narcan)

3. A nurse knows that teaching has been effective if a client who is taking a benzodiazepine for long-term treatment of anxiety states which of the following?

   A. "I will only take the medication at bedtime."

   B. "I will be able to keep taking this drug if I become pregnant."

   C. "I will not stop taking the drug abruptly."

   D. "I will need to take this medication the rest of my life."

4. A client has been taking buspirone (BuSpar) for 3 days to treat an anxiety disorder. He calls the community mental health facility and tells the nurse that the medication has not helped him to sleep at all, and that he is still feeling anxious. How should the nurse reply?

5. A client has been taking paroxetine (Paxil) to treat an anxiety disorder for several weeks. The client calls the nurse to say that he has been grinding his teeth during the night, which causes pain in his mouth and insomnia for his wife. Which of the following measures may be used to manage the client's concern? (Select all that apply.)

   _____ Concurrent administration of buspirone

   _____ Administration of a different SSRI

   _____ Use of a mouth guard

   _____ Changing to a different class of antianxiety medication

   _____ Increasing the dose of paroxetine

CHAPTER 19: MEDICATIONS FOR ANXIETY DISORDERS

 Application Exercises Answer Key

1. A nurse working in a mental health clinic is providing teaching to a client with a new prescription for diazepam (Valium) for generalized anxiety disorder. The client had originally told her provider that she took no other medications. However, before leaving the clinic, she says to the nurse, "Oh, I forgot that I do take a sleeping pill at night for insomnia, and I also usually drink a glass of wine before bedtime to make sure I sleep." What should be the nurse's concerns about this information, and what interventions are necessary?

Taking a benzodiazepine concurrently with other CNS depressants, including alcohol, can cause an overdose marked by increased sedation, lack of coordination, and confusion. This information should be reported to the provider before the client leaves the clinic.

 NCLEX® Connection: Pharmacological and Parenteral Therapies, Adverse Effects/ Contraindications/Side Effects/Interactions

2. Which of the following is an antidote for benzodiazepine overdose or toxicity?

    A. Buspirone (BuSpar)

    B. Venlafaxine (Effexor)

    C. Flumazenil (Romazicon)

    D. Naloxone (Narcan)

Flumazenil is a benzodiazepine receptor antagonist, which specifically reverses an overdose of benzodiazepines. Buspirone is a nonbarbiturate anxiolytic, and venlafaxine (Effexor) is an atypical antidepressant used for anxiety disorders. Naloxone is an opioid antagonist used to reverse an overdose of opioids, such as morphine sulfate.

 NCLEX® Connection: Pharmacological and Parenteral Therapies, Adverse Effects/ Contraindications/Side Effects/Interactions

3. A nurse knows that teaching has been effective if a client who is taking a benzodiazepine for long-term treatment of anxiety states which of the following?

    A. "I will only take the medication at bedtime."

    B. "I will be able to keep taking this drug if I become pregnant."

    C. "I will not stop taking the drug abruptly."

    D. "I will need to take this medication the rest of my life."

A client who takes a benzodiazepine over a long period of time may develop a physical dependence on the medication and may experience withdrawal symptoms if the medication is abruptly discontinued.

 NCLEX® Connection: Pharmacological and Parenteral Therapies, Medication Administration

4. A client has been taking buspirone (BuSpar) for 3 days to treat an anxiety disorder. He calls the community mental health facility and tells the nurse that the medication has not helped him to sleep at all, and that he is still feeling anxious. How should the nurse reply?

> **The initial response to buspirone takes 1 week, but it may take several weeks to reach its therapeutic peak. The medication has no hypnotic effect, so it does not promote sleep. Advise the client to try nonmedication measures to promote sleep.**

 NCLEX® Connection: Pharmacological and Parenteral Therapies, Expected Actions/ Outcomes

5. A client has been taking paroxetine (Paxil) to treat an anxiety disorder for several weeks. The client calls the nurse to say that he has been grinding his teeth during the night, which causes pain in his mouth and insomnia for his wife. Which of the following measures may be used to manage the client's concern? (Select all that apply.)

__X__	**Concurrent administration of buspirone**
_____	Administration of a different SSRI
__X__	**Use of a mouth guard**
__X__	**Changing to a different class of antianxiety medication**
_____	Increasing the dose of paroxetine

> **Concurrent administration of buspirone, use of a mouth guard, or changing to a different class of antianxiety medication are all ways to manage bruxism. Any SSRI may cause bruxism, so changing to another SSRI will not be effective. Increasing the dose of paroxetine will exacerbate the side effect.**

 NCLEX® Connection: Pharmacological and Parenteral Therapies, Adverse Effects/ Contraindications/Side Effects/Interactions

| UNIT 4 | PSYCHOPHARMACOLOGICAL THERAPIES |
| Chapter 20 | Medications for Depression |

Overview

- Depression is a mood (affective) disorder that is a widespread issue, ranking high among causes of disability.

- Clients starting antidepressant medication therapy for depression need to be advised that symptom relief can take 1 to 3 weeks, and possibly 2 to 3 months, for full therapeutic benefits to be reached. Encourage continued compliance.

- Clients diagnosed with major depression may require hospitalization with the implementation of close observation and suicide precautions until antidepressant medications reach their peak effect.

- Antidepressant medications are classified into four main groups:

  o Tricyclic antidepressants

  o Selective serotonin reuptake inhibitors (SSRIs)

  o Monoamine oxidase inhibitors (MAOIs)

  o Atypical antidepressants

MEDICATION CLASSIFICATION: TRICYCLIC ANTIDEPRESSANTS (TCAs)

- Select Prototype Medication: Amitriptyline (Elavil)

- Other Medications

  o Imipramine (Tofranil)

  o Doxepin (Sinequan)

  o Nortriptyline (Aventyl)

  o Amoxapine (Asendin)

  o Trimipramine (Surmontil)

Purpose

- Expected Pharmacological Action

  o These medications block reuptake of norepinephrine and serotonin in the synaptic space, thereby intensifying the effects of these neurotransmitters.

- Therapeutic Uses
  - Depression
  - Depressive episodes of bipolar disorders
- Other Uses
  - Chronic pain
  - Enuresis

Complications

SIDE/ADVERSE EFFECTS	NURSING INTERVENTIONS/CLIENT EDUCATION
Orthostatic hypotension	<ul><li>Instruct the client about the signs of postural hypotension (lightheadedness, dizziness). If these occur, advise the client to sit or lie down. Orthostatic hypotension can be minimized by getting up, or changing positions, slowly.</li><li>Monitor the hospitalized client's blood pressure and heart rate for orthostatic changes. If a significant decrease in blood pressure and/or increase in heart rate is noted, do not administer the medication, and notify the provider.</li></ul>
Anticholinergic effects • dry mouth • blurred vision • photophobia • urinary hesitancy or retention • constipation • tachycardia	<ul><li>Instruct the client on ways to minimize anticholinergic effects. These include:<ul><li>Chewing sugarless gum.</li><li>Sipping on water.</li><li>Wearing sunglasses when outdoors.</li><li>Eating foods high in fiber.</li><li>Exercising regularly.</li><li>Increasing fluid intake to at least 2 to 3 L/day from beverage and food sources.</li><li>Voiding just before taking the medication.</li></ul></li><li>Advise the client to notify the provider if symptoms persist.</li></ul>

SIDE/ADVERSE EFFECTS	NURSING INTERVENTIONS/CLIENT EDUCATION
Sedation	• This side effect usually diminishes over time. • Advise the clients to avoid hazardous activities, such as driving, if sedation is excessive. • Advise the client to take medication at bedtime to minimize daytime sleepiness and to promote sleep.
Toxicity resulting in cholinergic blockade and cardiac toxicity evidenced by dysrhythmias, mental confusion, and agitation, which are followed by seizures, coma, and possible death	• Give a 1-week supply of medication to clients who are acutely ill. • Obtain the client's baseline ECG. • Monitor vital signs frequently. • Monitor the client for signs of toxicity. • Notify the primary care provider if signs of toxicity occur.
Decreased seizure threshold	• Monitor clients who have seizure disorders.
Excessive sweating	• Inform the client of this side effect. Assist the client with frequent linen changes.

 Contraindications/Precautions

- Amitriptyline is a pregnancy risk category C medication.

- This medication is contraindicated for clients who have seizure disorders.

- Use this medication cautiously in clients with coronary artery disease; diabetes; liver, kidney and respiratory disorders; urinary retention and obstruction; angle closure glaucoma; benign prostatic hypertrophy; and hyperthyroidism.

Medication/Food interactions

MEDICATION/FOOD INTERACTIONS	NURSING INTERVENTIONS/CLIENT EDUCATION
Concurrent use with MAOIs may cause hypertension, which may become severe.	Avoid concurrent use of TCAs and MAOIs.
Concurrent use with antihistamines and other anticholinergic agents may result in additive anticholinergic effects.	Avoid concurrent use of TCAs and antihistamines.
Concurrent use with direct-acting sympathomimetics may result in increased effects of these medications, because uptake is blocked by TCAs.	Avoid concurrent use of TCAs and these medications.

MEDICATION/FOOD INTERACTIONS	NURSING INTERVENTIONS/CLIENT EDUCATION
Concurrent use with indirect-acting sympathomimetics may result in decreased effect of these medications, due to the inhibition of their uptake and inability to get to the site of action in the nerve terminal.	Avoid concurrent use of TCAs and these medications.
Concurrent use with alcohol, benzodiazepines, opioids, and antihistamines may result in additive CNS depression.	Advise the client to avoid other CNS depressants.

MEDICATION CLASSIFICATION: SELECTIVE SEROTONIN REUPTAKE INHIBITORS (SSRIs)

- Select Prototype Medication: Fluoxetine (Prozac)

- Other Medications

    o Citalopram (Celexa)

    o Escitalopram (Lexapro)

    o Paroxetine (Paxil)

    o Sertraline (Zoloft)

Purpose

- Expected Pharmacological Action

    o SSRIs selectively block reuptake of the monoamine neurotransmitter serotonin in the synaptic space, thereby intensifying the effects of serotonin.

- Therapeutic Uses

    o Major depression

    o Obsessive compulsive disorder

    o Bulimia nervosa

    o Premenstrual dysphoric disorders

    o Panic disorders

    o Posttraumatic disorder)

Complications

SIDE/ADVERSE EFFECTS	NURSING INTERVENTIONS/CLIENT EDUCATION
Sexual dysfunction (anorgasmia, impotence, decreased libido)	• Warn the client of possible side effects, and to notify the provider if they become intolerable. • Instruct the client on ways to manage sexual dysfunction, which may include lowering the dosage, discontinuing the medication temporarily (medication holiday), and using adjunct medications to improve sexual function. • Inform the client that an atypical antidepressant with fewer sexual dysfunction side effects (bupropion [Wellbutrin] and nefazodone [Serzone]) may be indicated.
CNS stimulation (inability to sleep, agitation, anxiety)	• Advise the client to notify the provider, as the dosage may need to be lowered. • Advise the client to take this medication in the morning • Advise the client to avoid caffeinated beverages • Teach the client relaxation techniques to promote sleep.
Occurrence of weight loss early in therapy that may be followed by weight gain with long-term treatment.	• Monitor the client's weight. • Encourage the client to participate in regular exercise and to follow a healthy, well-balanced diet.
Serotonin syndrome may begin 2 to 72 hr after the start of treatment, and it may be lethal. Manifestations include: • Mental confusion, difficulty concentrating • Agitation • Fever • Anxiety • Hallucinations • Hyperreflexia, incoordination • Diaphoresis • Tremors	• Advise the client to observe for symptoms. If symptoms occur, instruct the client to discontinue the medication and notify the provider.
Withdrawal syndrome (headache, nausea, visual disturbances, anxiety, dizziness, and tremors)	• Instruct the client to taper the dose gradually when discontinuing the medication.

SIDE/ADVERSE EFFECTS	NURSING INTERVENTIONS/CLIENT EDUCATION
Hyponatremia, which is more likely to occur in older adult clients taking diuretics	• Obtain a baseline serum sodium, and monitor the level periodically throughout treatment.
Rash	• Advise the client that a rash can be treated with an antihistamine or withdrawal from the medication.
Sleepiness, faintness, lightheadedness	• Advise the client that these side effects are not common, but can occur. • The client should avoid driving if these side effects occur.
Gastrointestinal bleeding	• Use cautiously in clients with a history of gastrointestinal bleeding, ulcers, and those taking other medications that affect blood coagulation.
Bruxism	• Advise the client to report this to the provider. • Advise the client to use a mouth guard, and that changing to a different classification of antidepressants, or adding a low dose of buspirone, may be indicated.

 Contraindications/Precautions

- Fluoxetine is a pregnancy risk category C medication.

- Fluoxetine and paroxetine may increase the risk of birth defects. Other SSRIs should be used. Late in pregnancy, use of SSRIs may increase the risk of withdrawal symptoms or pulmonary hypertension in the newborn.

- These medications are contraindicated in clients taking MAOIs or TCAs.

- Use cautiously in clients with liver and/or renal dysfunction, cardiac disease, seizure disorders, diabetes, ulcers, and a history of gastrointestinal bleeding.

Medication/Food interactions

MEDICATION/FOOD INTERACTIONS	NURSING INTERVENTIONS/CLIENT EDUCATION
Concurrent use with MAOIs, TCAs, St. John's Wort increases the risk of serotonin syndrome.	• MAOIs should be discontinued for 14 days prior to starting an SSRI. Fluoxetine should be discontinued 5 weeks before starting an MAOI. • Advise the client against concurrent use of TCAs and St. John's Wort.

MEDICATION/FOOD INTERACTIONS	NURSING INTERVENTIONS/CLIENT EDUCATION
Concurrent use with warfarin (Coumadin) can displace warfarin from bound protein and result in increased warfarin levels.	• Monitor the client's prothrombin time (PTT) and INR levels. • Assess the client for signs of bleeding and the need for dosage adjustment.
Concurrent use with tricyclic antidepressants and lithium may result in increased levels of these medications.	• Advise the client to avoid concurrent use.
Concurrent use with NSAIDs and anticoagulants can further suppress platelet aggregation, thereby increasing the risk of bleeding.	• Advise the client to monitor for signs of bleeding (bruising, hematuria) and to notify the provider if they occur.

MEDICATION CLASSIFICATION: MONOAMINE OXIDASE INHIBITORS (MAOIs)

- Select Prototype Medication: Phenelzine (Nardil)

- Other Medications

  o Isocarboxazid (Marplan)

  o Tranylcypromine (Parnate)

  o Selegiline (Emsam) – transdermal patch

Purpose

- Expected Pharmacological Action

  o These medications block MAO-A in the brain, thereby increasing the amount of norepinephrine, dopamine, and serotonin available for transmission of impulses. An increased amount of those neurotransmitters at nerve endings intensifies responses and relieves depression.

- Therapeutic Uses

  o Atypical depression

  o Bulimia nervosa

  o Obsessive compulsive disorder

Complications

SIDE/ADVERSE EFFECTS	NURSING INTERVENTIONS/CLIENT EDUCATION
CNS stimulation (e.g., anxiety, agitation, hypomania, mania)	• Advise the client to observe for symptoms and to notify the provider if they occur.

SIDE/ADVERSE EFFECTS	NURSING INTERVENTIONS/CLIENT EDUCATION
Orthostatic hypotension	• Monitor the client's blood pressure and heart rate for orthostatic changes. • Hold the medication, and notify the provider regarding significant changes. • Advise the client to change positions slowly.
Hypertensive crisis resulting from intake of dietary tyramine – severe hypertension as a result of intensive vasoconstriction and stimulation of the heart. Manifestations may include: • Headache • Nausea • Increased heart rate • Increased blood pressure	• Administer phentolamine (Regitine) IV, a rapid-acting alpha-adrenergic blocker, or nifedipine (Procardia). • Provide continuous cardiac monitoring and respiratory support as indicated.
Local rash associated with transdermal preparation	• Choose a clean, dry area for each application. • Apply a topical glucocorticoid on the affected areas if rash occurs.

 Contraindications/Precautions

- Phenelzine is a pregnancy risk category C medication.

- MAOIs are contraindicated in clients taking SSRIs, or clients with pheochromocytoma, heart failure, cardiovascular and cerebral vascular disease, and/or severe renal insufficiency.

- Use cautiously in clients with diabetes and/or seizure disorders, or those taking TCAs.

- Transdermal selegiline is contraindicated for clients taking carbamazepine (Tegretol) or oxcarbazepine (Trileptal). Concurrent use of these medications may increase blood levels of the MAOI.

Medication/Food interactions

MEDICATION/FOOD INTERACTIONS	NURSING INTERVENTIONS/CLIENT EDUCATION
Concurrent use with indirect-acting sympathomimetic medications (ephedrine, amphetamine) can promote the release of norepinephrine and lead to hypertensive crisis.	• Instruct the client that over-the-counter decongestants and cold remedies frequently contain medications with sympathomimetic action and should therefore be avoided.
Concurrent use with TCAs can lead to hypertensive crisis.	• Concurrent use of MAOIs and TCAs should be implemented cautiously.

MEDICATION/FOOD INTERACTIONS	NURSING INTERVENTIONS/CLIENT EDUCATION
Concurrent use with SSRIs can lead to serotonin syndrome.	• Avoid concurrent use.
Concurrent use with antihypertensives may cause additive hypotensive effects.	• Monitor the client's blood pressure. • Notify the provider if there is a significant drop in the client's blood pressure, as the dosage of antihypertensive may need to be reduced.
Concurrent use with meperidine (Demerol) can lead to hyperpyrexia.	• Alternative analgesic should be used.
Hypertensive crisis (severe hypertension as a result of intensive vasoconstriction and stimulation of the heart) can result from intake of dietary tyramine. Manifestations may include: • Headache • Nausea • Increase heart rate • Increased blood pressure	• Assess the client for ability to follow strict adherence to dietary restrictions. • Inform the client of symptoms and to notify the primary care provider if they occur. • Provide the client with written instructions regarding foods and beverages to be avoided. • Tyramine-rich foods include aged cheese, pepperoni, salami, avocados, figs, bananas, smoked fish, protein, some dietary supplements, some beers, and red wine. • Advise the client to avoid taking any medications without approval from the provider.
Concurrent use with vasopressors (caffeine, phenylethylamine) may result in hypertension.	• Advise the client to avoid foods that contain these agents (caffeinated beverages, chocolate, fava beans, ginseng).

MEDICATION CLASSIFICATION: ATYPICAL ANTIDEPRESSANTS

- Select Prototype Medication: Bupropion (Wellbutrin)

Purpose

- Expected Pharmacological Action

  o This medication acts by inhibiting dopamine uptake.

- Therapeutic Uses

  o Treatment of depression

  o Alternative to SSRIs for clients unable to tolerate the sexual dysfunction side effects

  o Aid to quit smoking

  o Prevention of seasonal affective disorder

Complications

SIDE/ADVERSE EFFECTS	NURSING INTERVENTIONS/CLIENT EDUCATION
Headache, dry mouth, GI distress, constipation, increased heart rate, nausea, restlessness, insomnia	• Advise the client to observe for symptoms and to notify the provider if they become intolerable. • Treat headaches with a mild analgesic. • Advise the client to sip fluids to treat dry mouth, and to increase dietary fiber to prevent constipation.
Suppression of appetite resulting in weight loss	• Monitor the client's food intake and weight.
Seizures, especially at higher dose ranges	• Avoid administering to clients at risk for seizures, such as a client with a head injury. • Monitor clients for seizures, and treat accordingly.

Ⓢ Contraindications/Precautions

- Bupropion is a pregnancy risk category B medication.

- This medication should be used cautiously in clients with a seizure disorder.

- This medication is contraindicated in clients taking MAOIs.

Medication/Food interactions

MEDICATION/FOOD INTERACTIONS	NURSING INTERVENTIONS/CLIENT EDUCATION
Concurrent use with MAOIs, such as phenelzine (Nardil), may increase the risk for toxicity.	• MAOIs should be discontinued 2 weeks prior to beginning treatment with bupropion.

OTHER ATYPICAL ANTIDEPRESSANTS

AGENT	PHARMACOLOGICAL ACTION	NURSING IMPLICATIONS
Venlafaxine (Effexor), duloxetine (Cymbalta)	These agents inhibit serotonin and norepinephrine reuptake, thereby increasing the amount of these neurotransmitters available in the brain for impulse transmission. There is also a minimal amount of dopamine blockade.	• Side effects include headache, nausea, agitation, anxiety, and sleep disturbances. • Monitor for hyponatremia, especially in older adult clients. • Monitor the client for weight loss. • Monitor the client for increases in diastolic blood pressure. • Discuss ways to manage interference with sexual functioning. • Advise the client to avoid abrupt cessation of the medication.
Mirtazapine (Remeron)	This agent increases the release of serotonin and norepinephrine, thereby increasing the amount of these neurotransmitters available for impulse transmission.	• Therapeutic effects may occur sooner, and with less sexual dysfunction, than with SSRIs. • This medication is generally well tolerated. Side effects include sleepiness that can be exacerbated by other CNS depressants, weight gain, and elevated cholesterol.
Reboxetine (Edronax)	This agent selectively inhibits the reuptake of norepinephrine, thereby increasing the amount of neurotransmitters available for impulse transmission.	• This medication yields similar results as SSRIs. • Reboxetine is generally well tolerated, but clients may experience dry mouth, decreased blood pressure, constipation, sexual dysfunction, and urinary hesitancy or retention. • Weight gain and sleepiness do not occur with this medication. • Avoid concurrent use with an MAOI.
Trazodone (Desyrel)	This agent has moderate selective blockade of serotonin receptors, thereby increasing the amount of that neurotransmitter available for impulse transmission.	• This agent is usually used with another antidepressant agent. Sedation may be an issue; therefore, it may be indicated for a client with insomnia caused by an SSRI. • Priapism may be a serious side effect, and clients should be instructed to seek medical attention immediately if this occurs.

Nursing Administration

- Instruct the client to take this medication as prescribed on a daily basis to establish therapeutic plasma levels.

- Assist with the client's medication regimen compliance by informing the client that therapeutic effects may not be experienced for 1 to 3 weeks. Full therapeutic effects may take 2 to 3 months.

- Instruct the client to continue therapy after improvement in symptoms. Sudden discontinuation of the medication can result in relapse.

- Advise the client that therapy usually continues for 6 months after resolution of symptoms, and it may continue for a year or longer.

Ⓢ - Suicide prevention can be facilitated by prescribing only a week's worth of medication for an acutely ill client, and then only prescribing 1 month's worth of medication at a time, especially with TCAs.

- For SSRIs:

    o Advise clients to take these medications in the morning to minimize sleep disturbances.

    o Advise clients to take these medications with food to minimize gastrointestinal disturbances.

Ⓖ o Obtain baseline sodium levels for older adult client taking diuretics; monitor these clients periodically.

Nursing Evaluation of Medication Effectiveness

- Depending on therapeutic intent, effectiveness may be evidenced by:

    o Verbalizing improvement in mood.

    o Ability to perform ADLs

    o Improved sleeping and eating habits.

    o Increased interaction with peers

CHAPTER 20: MEDICATIONS FOR DEPRESSION

 Application Exercises

1. A nurse is providing teaching to a client with a new prescription for amitriptyline (Elavil). Which of the following client statements indicates understanding of the teaching?

    A. "I should stay out of the sun to prevent getting a skin rash."

    B. "I may feel drowsy for a few weeks after starting this medication."

    C. "I cannot eat my favorite pizza with pepperoni anymore."

    D. "I will finally be able to lose the weight that I have gained over the last year."

2. A nurse is caring for a client who is taking phenelzine (Nardil). For which of the following side effects should the nurse observe? (Select all that apply.)

    _____ Elevated blood glucose level

    _____ Orthostatic hypotension

    _____ Rash

    _____ Headache

    _____ Bruxism

3. A client has been prescribed bupropion (Wellbutrin) for depression. Upon reviewing the client's chart, the nurse should report which of the following findings to the client's provider immediately?

    A. The client has a family history of depression.

    B. The client swims three times a week for exercise.

    C. The client had a motor vehicle crash last year and sustained a head injury.

    D. The client has been dieting and has lost 10 pounds over the last year.

4. Which of the following antidepressants increases the release of serotonin and norepinephrine?

    A. Mirtazapine (Remeron)

    B. Venlafaxine (Effexor)

    C. Trazodone (Desyrel)

    D. Imipramine (Tofranil)

CHAPTER 20: MEDICATIONS FOR DEPRESSION

 Application Exercises Answer Key

1. A nurse is providing teaching to a client with a new prescription for amitriptyline (Elavil). Which of the following client statements indicates understanding of the teaching?

    A. "I should stay out of the sun to prevent getting a skin rash."

    B. "I may feel drowsy for a few weeks after starting this medication."

    C. "I cannot eat my favorite pizza with pepperoni anymore."

    D. "I will finally be able to lose the weight that I have gained over the last year."

Sedation is a side effect of amitriptyline (Elavil) during the first few weeks of therapy. Usually this is self-limiting. Skin rash is more likely to occur with fluoxetine. Foods such as pepperoni should be avoided if the client is prescribed a monoamine oxidase inhibitor. Weight gain, rather than weight loss is expected with TCAs.

 NCLEX® Connection: Pharmacological and Parenteral Therapies, Adverse Effects/ Contraindications/Side Effects/Interactions

2. A nurse is caring for a client who is taking phenelzine (Nardil). For which of the following side effects should the nurse observe? (Select all that apply.)

    _____ Elevated blood glucose level

    __**X**__ **Orthostatic hypotension**

    _____ Rash

    __**X**__ **Headache**

    _____ Bruxism

Orthostatic hypotension and headache are side effects for which the nurse should observe. Phenelzine does not result in elevated blood glucose levels, and a rash is associated with transdermal preparations. Bruxism is a side effect common with fluoxetine.

 NCLEX® Connection: Pharmacological and Parenteral Therapies, Adverse Effects/ Contraindications/Side Effects/Interactions

3. A client has been prescribed bupropion (Wellbutrin) for depression. Upon reviewing the client's chart, the nurse should report which of the following findings to the client's provider immediately?

    A. The client has a family history of depression.

    B. The client swims three times a week for exercise.

    C. The client had a motor vehicle crash last year and sustained a head injury.

    D. The client has been dieting and has lost 10 pounds over the last year.

The greatest risk to this client is development of seizures. Bupropion can lower the seizure threshold and should be avoided by clients with a history of a head injury. The client's family history of depression, usual activities, and current nutritional status are important but do not need to be reported to the provider immediately.

 NCLEX® Connection: Pharmacological and Parenteral Therapies, Adverse Effects/ Contraindications/Side Effects/Interactions

4. Which of the following antidepressants increases the release of serotonin and norepinephrine?

   A. Mirtazapine (Remeron)

   B. Venlafaxine (Effexor)

   C. Trazodone (Desyrel)

   D. Imipramine (Tofranil)

   Mirtazapine increases the release of serotonin and norepinephrine, and thereby increases the amount available in the brain for impulse transmission. Venlafaxine is a serotonin/ norepinephrine reuptake inhibitor. Trazodone is an atypical antidepressant that results in moderate blockade of serotonin. Imipramine is a TCA that blocks the reuptake of norepinephrine and serotonin.

   Ⓝ **NCLEX® Connection: Pharmacological and Parenteral Therapies, Expected Actions/ Outcomes**

UNIT 4	PSYCHOPHARMACOLOGICAL THERAPIES
Chapter 21	Medications for Bipolar Disorders

Overview

- Bipolar disorder is primarily managed with mood stabilizing medications, such as lithium carbonate (Lithane, Eskalith, Lithobid).

- Bipolar disorder can also be treated with certain antiepileptic medications, such as:

  o Valproic acid (Depakote)

  o Carbamazepine (Tegretol)

  o Lamotrigine (Lamictal)

- Other medications used for bipolar disorder include:

  o Atypical antipsychotics – These can be useful in early treatment to promote sleep and to decrease anxiety and agitation. These medications also demonstrate mood-stabilizing properties.

  o Anxiolytics – Clonazepam (Klonopin) and lorazepam (Ativan) can be useful in treating acute mania and managing the psychomotor agitation often seen in mania.

MEDICATION CLASSIFICATION: MOOD STABILIZER

- Select Prototype Medication: Lithium Carbonate

Purpose

- Expected Pharmacological Action

  o Lithium produces neurochemical changes in the brain, including serotonin receptor blockade.

  o There is evidence that lithium decreases neuronal atrophy and/or increases neuronal growth.

- Therapeutic Uses

  o Lithium is used in the treatment of bipolar disorders. Lithium controls episodes of acute mania, helps to prevent the return of mania or depression, and decreases the incidence of suicide.

  o Other uses include:

    ▪ Alcoholism

    ▪ Bulimia

    ▪ Schizophrenia

Complications

- Effects of Therapeutic Lithium Levels (Some effects will resolve within a few weeks.)

SIDE/ADVERSE EFFECTS	NURSING INTERVENTIONS/CLIENT EDUCATION
Gastrointestinal distress (nausea, diarrhea, abdominal pain)	• Advise the client that symptoms are usually transient. • Administer medication with meals or milk.
Fine hand tremors that can interfere with purposeful motor skills and can be exacerbated by factors such as stress and caffeine	• Administer beta-adrenergic blocking agents such as propranolol (Inderal). • Adjust dosage to be as low as possible, give in divided doses, or use long-acting formulations. • Advise the client to report an increase in tremors, which could be a sign of lithium toxicity.
Polyuria, mild thirst	• Use a potassium-sparing diuretic, such as spironolactone (Aldactone). • Instruct the client to maintain adequate fluid intake by consuming at least 2,000 to 3,000 mL of fluid/day from beverages or food sources.
Weight gain	• Assist the client to follow a healthy diet and regular exercise regimen
Renal toxicity	• Monitor the client's I&O. • Adjust dosage, and keep dose at the lowest level necessary. • Assess baseline BUN and creatinine, and monitor kidney function periodically.
Goiter and hypothyroidism with long-term treatment	• Obtain the client's baseline T_3, T_4, and TSH levels prior to starting treatment, and then annually. • Advise the client to monitor for signs of hypothyroidism (cold, dry skin; decreased heart rate, weight gain). • Administer levothyroxine (Synthroid) to manage hyperthyroidism.
Bradydysrhythmias, hypotension, electrolyte imbalances	• Encourage the client to maintain adequate fluid intake.

SIGNS AND SYMPTOMS OF TOXICITY			
Early signs	Less than 1.5 mEq/L	Diarrhea, nausea, vomiting, thirst, polyuria, muscle weakness and slurred speech	• Instruct the client to discontinue the medication, and notify the provider. • Administer new dosage based on the client's serum lithium levels.

SIGNS AND SYMPTOMS OF TOXICITY			
Advanced signs	1.5 to 2.0 mEq/L	Mental confusion, poor coordination, coarse tremors, and ongoing gastrointestinal distress including nausea, vomiting, and diarrhea	• Instruct the client to discontinue the medication, and notify the provider. • Administer new dosage based on the client's serum sodium levels. • Excretion may need to be promoted.
Severe toxicity	Greater than 2.0 to 2.5 mEq/L	Extreme polyuria of dilute urine, tinnitus, blurred vision, ataxia, seizures, severe hypotension leading to coma, and possible death from respiratory complications	• Administer an emetic to alert clients, or administer gastric lavage. • Urea, mannitol, or aminophylline may be prescribed to increase the rate of excretion.
	Greater than 2.5 mEq/L	Rapid progression of symptoms leading to coma and death	• Hemodialysis may be warranted.

Ⓢ Contraindications/Precautions

- Lithium is a pregnancy risk category D medication. It is considered teratogenic, especially during the first trimester of pregnancy.

- Discourage clients from breastfeeding if lithium therapy is necessary.

- Use cautiously in clients with renal dysfunction, heart disease, sodium depletion, and dehydration.

Medication/Food Interactions

MEDICATION/FOOD INTERACTIONS	NURSING INTERVENTIONS/CLIENT EDUCATION
Diuretics – Sodium is excreted with the use of diuretics; with decreased serum sodium, lithium excretion is decreased , which can lead to toxicity.	• Monitor the client for signs of toxicity. • Advise the client to observe for symptoms and to notify the provider. • Encourage the client to maintain a diet adequate in sodium, and to drink 2,000 mL to 3,000 mL of water/day.
NSAIDs (ibuprofen [Motrin] and celecoxib [Celebrex]) – concurrent use will increase renal reabsorption of lithium, leading to toxicity.	• Avoid use of NSAIDs to prevent toxic accumulation of lithium. • Use aspirin as a mild analgesic.
Anticholinergics (antihistamines, tricyclic antidepressants) – abdominal discomfort can result from anticholinergic-induced urinary retention and polyuria.	• Advise the client to avoid medications with anticholinergic effects.

Nursing Administration

- Monitor plasma lithium levels while undergoing treatment. At initiation of treatment, monitor levels every 2 to 3 days until stable, and then every 1 to 3 months. Lithium blood levels should be obtained in the morning, usually 12 hr after last dose.

    o During initial treatment of a manic episode, levels should be between 0.8 to 1.4 mEq/L.

    o Maintenance level range is between 0.4 to 1.0 mEq/L.

    o Plasma levels > 1.5 mEq/L can result in toxicity.

- Care for a client with a toxic plasma lithium level should take place in an inpatient setting and supportive measures provided. Hemodialysis may be indicated.

- Advise the client that effects begin within 7 to 14 days.

- Advise the client to take lithium as prescribed. This medication must be administered in 2 to 3 doses daily, due to a short half-life. Taking lithium with food will help decrease GI distress.

- Encourage the client to adhere to laboratory appointments needed to monitor lithium effectiveness and adverse effects. Emphasize the high risk of toxicity due to the narrow therapeutic range.

- Provide nutritional counseling. Stress the importance of adequate fluid and sodium intake.

- Instruct the client to monitor for signs of toxicity and when to contact the provider. The client should stop taking medication and seek medical attention if she is experiencing diarrhea, vomiting, or excessive sweating.

MEDICATION CLASSIFICATION: MOOD-STABILIZING ANTIEPILEPTIC DRUGS (AEDs)

- Select Prototype Medications:

    o Carbamazepine (Tegretol)

    o Valproic acid (Depakote)

    o Lamotrigine (Lamictal)

Purpose

- Expected Pharmacological Action

    o AEDs help treat and manage bipolar disorder through various mechanisms, which include:

        ▪ Slowing the entrance of sodium and calcium back into the neuron, thus extending the time it takes for the nerve to return to its active state

        ▪ Potentiating the inhibitory effects of gamma butyric acid (GABA)

        ▪ Inhibiting glutamic acid (glutamate), which in turn suppresses CNS excitation

- Therapeutic Uses

  o These medications are used to treat manic and depressive episodes, as well as to prevent relapse of mania and depressive episodes. They are particularly useful for clients with mixed mania and rapid cycling bipolar disorders.

Complications

SIDE/ADVERSE EFFECTS	NURSING INTERVENTIONS/CLIENT EDUCATION
Carbamazepine (Tegretol)	

• Minimal effect on cognitive function
• CNS effects:
  o Nystagmus
  o Double vision
  o Vertigo
  o Staggering gait
  o Headache
	• Administer in low doses initially, and then gradually increase dosage.
	• Advise the client that symptoms should subside within a few weeks.
	• Administer dose at bedtime.

• Blood dyscrasias (leukopenia, anemia, thrombocytopenia)	• Obtain the client's baseline CBC and platelets. Perform ongoing monitoring of these. • Observe the client for signs of bruising and bleeding of gums.
• Teratogenesis	• Advise the client to avoid use in pregnancy.
Hypo-osmolarity – promotes secretion of ADH, which inhibits water excretion by the kidneys, and places the client with heart failure at risk for fluid overload	• Monitor the client's serum sodium. • Monitor the client for edema, decrease in urine output, and hypertension.
Skin disorders include dermatitis, rash (Stevens-Johnson syndrome)	• Treat mild reactions with anti-inflammatory or antihistamine medications. • Advise the client to wear sunscreen. • Instruct the client to discontinue the medication, and notify the provider if Stevens-Johnson rash occurs.

SIDE/ADVERSE EFFECTS	NURSING INTERVENTIONS/CLIENT EDUCATION
Valproic Acid (Depakote)	
Gastrointestinal effects include nausea, vomiting, and indigestion	• Advise the client that these symptoms are generally self-limiting • Advise the client to take medication with food, or switch to enteric-coated formulations.
Hepatotoxicity as evidence by anorexia, nausea, vomiting, fatigue, abdominal pain, jaundice	• Assess baseline liver function, and monitor liver function regularly. • Advise the client to observe for signs and symptoms of hepatotoxicity and to notify the provider immediately if they occur. • Avoid using in children younger than 2 years old. • Administer the lowest effective dose.
Pancreatitis as evidenced by nausea, vomiting, abdominal pain	• Advise the client to observe for signs and symptoms of pancreatitis and to notify the provider immediately if they occur. • Monitor the client's amylase levels. • Discontinue the medication if pancreatitis develops.
Thrombocytopenia	• Advise the client to observe for signs and symptoms, such as bruising and to notify the provider if these occur. • Monitor the client's platelet counts.
Teratogenesis	• Advise the client to avoid use during pregnancy.
Lamotrigine (Lamictal)	
Double or blurred vision, dizziness, headache, nausea, vomiting	• Caution the client about performing activities that require concentration.
Serious skin rashes, including Stevens-Johnson syndrome	• Instruct the client to discontinue the medication, and notify the provider if a rash occurs.

Ⓢ Contraindications/Precautions

- These medications are pregnancy risk category D medications, as they can result in birth defects.

- Carbamazepine is contraindicated in clients with bone marrow suppression or with bleeding disorders.

- Valproic acid is contraindicated in clients with liver disorders.

Medication/Food Interactions

MEDICATION/FOOD INTERACTIONS	NURSING INTERVENTIONS/CLIENT EDUCATION
Carbamazepine (Tegretol)	
Oral contraceptives, warfarin (Coumadin): concurrent use of carbamazepine causes a decrease in the effects of these medications, due to stimulation of hepatic and drug-metabolizing enzymes.	• Advise the client to use an alternate form of birth control. • Monitor for therapeutic effects of warfarin. Dosage may need to be adjusted.
Grapefruit juice: inhibits metabolism of carbamazepine, thereby increasing blood levels of the medication.	Advise the client to avoid all intake of grapefruit juice.
Phenytoin, phenobarbital: concurrent use decreases the effects of carbamazepine by stimulating metabolism.	Monitor phenytoin and phenobarbital levels, and adjust dosages as prescribed.
Valproic Acid (Depakote)	
Phenytoin, phenobarbital: concurrent use increases the levels of these medications.	Monitor phenytoin and phenobarbital levels, and adjust dosages as prescribed.
Lamotrigine (Lamictal)	
Carbamazepine, phenytoin, phenobarbital: concurrent use promotes liver drug-metabolizing enzymes, thereby decreasing the effect of lamotrigine.	Monitor for therapeutic effects, and adjust dosages as prescribed.
Valproic acid: concurrent use inhibits drug-metabolizing enzymes, thereby increasing the half-life of lamotrigine.	Monitor for adverse effects, and adjust dosages as prescribed.

Nursing Evaluation of Medication Effectiveness

- Depending on therapeutic intent, effectiveness may be evidenced by:
    - Relief of acute manic symptoms (flight of ideas, obsessive talking, agitation) or depressive symptoms (fatigue, poor appetite, psychomotor retardation)
    - Verbalization of improvement in mood
    - Ability to perform ADLs
    - Improved sleeping and eating habits
    - Greater interaction with peers

CHAPTER 21: MEDICATIONS FOR BIPOLAR DISORDERS

 Application Exercises

1. A client who has been on lithium therapy for 6 months has recently developed symptoms of mild arthritis. He tells the nurse that he wants to start taking ibuprofen for his pain. Which of the following is an appropriate response?

    A. "That is a good choice. Stronger analgesics would not be good for you."

    B. "Regular aspirin would be a better choice, because ibuprofen can raise your lithium level too high."

    C. "You will have to stop taking the lithium if you take any pain medication."

    D. "The ibuprofen will make your lithium level fall too low, and your symptoms may return."

2. A client is started on valproic acid (Depakote) for treatment of bipolar disorder. Which of the following laboratory studies should be monitored regularly?

    A. AST/ALT and LDH

    B. Creatinine and BUN

    C. WBC and granulocyte counts

    D. Serum sodium and potassium

3. Which of the following medications, if given concurrently with lithium, could produce a toxic effect?

    A. Insulin

    B. Prednisone

    C. Digoxin (Lanoxin)

    D. Furosemide (Lasix)

4. A nurse is providing teaching to a client prescribed lithium carbonate for bipolar disorder. For which of the following side effects should the nurse instruct the client to watch and report to the provider? (Select all that apply.)

    _____   Constipation

    _____   Polyuria

    _____   Rash

    _____   Muscle weakness

    _____   Weight loss

CHAPTER 21: MEDICATIONS FOR BIPOLAR DISORDERS

 Application Exercises Answer Key

1. A client who has been on lithium therapy for 6 months has recently developed symptoms of mild arthritis. He tells the nurse that he wants to start taking ibuprofen for his pain. Which of the following is an appropriate response?

   A. "That is a good choice. Stronger analgesics would not be good for you."

   B. "Regular aspirin would be a better choice, because ibuprofen can raise your lithium level too high."

   C. "You will have to stop taking the lithium if you take any pain medication."

   D. "The ibuprofen will make your lithium level fall too low, and your symptoms may return."

   Ibuprofen increases renal lithium reabsorption; aspirin does not increase lithium levels. Stronger analgesics are not necessary for mild arthritis. Not all pain medications are contraindicated with concurrent use of lithium. Ibuprofen will not make the lithium level fall too low.

    NCLEX® Connection: Pharmacological and Parenteral Therapies, Adverse Effects/ Contraindications/Side Effects/Interactions

2. A client is started on valproic acid (Depakote) for treatment of bipolar disorder. Which of the following laboratory studies should be monitored regularly?

   A. AST/ALT and LDH

   B. Creatinine and BUN

   C. WBC and granulocyte counts

   D. Serum sodium and potassium

   Liver function tests should be monitored, because valproic acid is metabolized in the liver, and hepatotoxicity may result. Baseline levels may be drawn for creatinine and BUN (kidney function tests), WBC and granulocyte counts (tests to monitor for infection), or serum sodium and potassium (electrolytes), but regular monitoring of these values is not necessary.

   NCLEX® Connection: Pharmacological and Parenteral Therapies, Adverse Effects/ Contraindications/Side Effects/Interactions

3. Which of the following medications, if given concurrently with lithium, could produce a toxic effect?

   A. Insulin

   B. Prednisone

   C. Digoxin (Lanoxin)

   D. Furosemide (Lasix)

   Furosemide, a loop diuretic, promotes sodium loss and lithium retention, possibly increasing serum levels. Insulin, prednisone, and digoxin do not interact with lithium.

   NCLEX® Connection: Pharmacological and Parenteral Therapies, Adverse Effects/ Contraindications/Side Effects/Interactions

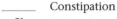

4. A nurse is providing teaching to a client prescribed lithium carbonate for bipolar disorder. For which of the following side effects should the nurse instruct the client to watch and report to the provider? (Select all that apply.)

    _____   Constipation

    __**X**__   **Polyuria**

    _____   Rash

    __**X**__   **Muscle weakness**

    _____   Weight loss

Polyuria and muscle weakness are early indications of lithium toxicity. The client is more likely to have diarrhea and weight gain, and a rash is not a sign of lithium toxicity.

 NCLEX® Connection: Pharmacological and Parenteral Therapies, Adverse Effects/Contraindications/Side Effects/Interactions

Overview

- Schizophrenia is the primary reason for the administration of antipsychotic medications.

  - The clinical course of schizophrenia usually involves acute exacerbations with intervals of semiremission.

  - Medications are used to treat:

    - Positive symptoms related to behavior, thought, and speech (agitation, delusions, hallucinations, tangential speech patterns)

    - Negative symptoms (social withdrawal, lack of emotion, lack of energy, flattened affect, decreased motivation, decreased pleasure in activities).The goals of psychopharmacological treatment for schizophrenia include:

      - Suppression of acute episodes

      - Prevention of acute recurrence

      - Maintenance of the highest possible level of functioning

- Conventional antipsychotic medications are used mainly to control positive symptoms of psychosis and are reserved for clients who are

  - Using them successfully and can tolerate the side effects.

  - Violent or particularly aggressive.

- Atypical antipsychotic agents are now medications of choice for clients receiving initial treatment, and for treating breakthrough episodes in clients on conventional medication therapy, because they are more effective with fewer adverse effects.

  - Advantages of atypical antipsychotic agents include:

    - Relief of both positive and negative symptoms

    - Decrease in affective symptoms (depression, anxiety) and suicidal behaviors

    - Improvement of neurocognitive defects, such as poor memory

    - Fewer or no extrapyramidal symptoms (EPS), including tardive dyskinesia, due to less dopamine blockade

    - Fewer anticholinergic effects, with the exception of clozapine (Clozaril), which has a high incidence of anticholinergic effects. This is because most of the atypical antipsychotics cause little or no blockade of cholinergic receptors

    - Less relapse

MEDICATION CLASSIFICATION: ANTIPSYCHOTICS - CONVENTIONAL

- Select Prototype Medication: Chlorpromazine (Thorazine):

- Other Medications

  - Haloperidol (Haldol), high potency

  - Fluphenazine (Prolixin), high potency

  - Molindone (Moban), medium potency

  - Loxapine (Loxitane), medium potency

  - Thioridazine (Mellaril), low potency

  - Thiothixene (Navane), high potency

Purpose

- Expected Pharmacological Action

  - The conventional antipsychotic medications block dopamine (D_2), acetylcholine, histamine, and norepinephrine (NE) receptors in the brain and periphery.

  - Inhibition of psychotic symptoms is believed to be a result of D_2 blockade in the brain.

- Therapeutic Uses

  - Treatment of acute and chronic psychosis

  - Schizophrenia

  - Bipolar disorder – primarily the manic phase

  - Tourette's syndrome

  - Delusional and schizoaffective disorder

  - Dementia

  - Prevention of nausea/vomiting through blocking of dopamine in the chemoreceptor trigger zone of the medulla

Complications

SIDE/ADVERSE EFFECTS	NURSING INTERVENTIONS/CLIENT EDUCATION
Acute dystonia • Severe spasm of the tongue, neck, face, and back • Crisis situation that requires rapid treatment	• Begin to monitor for side effects anywhere between 5 hr to 5 days after administration of first dose. • Treat these side effects with anticholinergic agents, such as benztropine (Cogentin) or diphenhydramine (Benadryl).
Parkinsonism • Bradykinesia • Rigidity • Shuffling gait • Drooling • Tremors	• Observe for signs and symptoms for the first month after the initiation of therapy. • Treat these side effects with benztropine, diphenhydramine, or amantadine (Symmetrel).
Akathisia • Inability to sit or stand still • Continual pacing and agitation	• Observe for signs and symptoms for the first 2 months after the initiation of treatment. • Manage symptoms with beta-blockers, benzodiazepines, or anticholinergic medications.

Late extrapyramidal side effects
• Tardive dyskinesia
  ○ Involuntary movements of the tongue and face, such as lip smacking
  ○ Involuntary movements of the arms, legs, and trunk
	• Administer lowest dosage possible to control symptoms.
	• Evaluate the client after 12 months of therapy and then every 3 months. Manifestations may occur months to years after the initiation of therapy. If signs of TD appear, dosage should be lowered, or the client should be switched to an atypical agent.
	• Use the Abnormal Involuntary Movement Scale (AIMS) to screen for the presence of EPS.

Neuroleptic malignant syndrome • Sudden high fever • Blood pressure fluctuations • Dysrhythmias • Muscle rigidity • Changes in level of consciousness • Coma	• Stop antipsychotic medication. • Monitor the client's vital signs. • Apply cooling blankets. • Administer antipyretics, such as aspirin or acetaminophen. • Increase the client's fluid intake. • Administer dantrolene (Dantrium) and bromocriptine (Parlodel) to induce muscle relaxation. • Wait 2 weeks before resuming therapy. Consider switching to an atypical agent.

SIDE/ADVERSE EFFECTS	NURSING INTERVENTIONS/CLIENT EDUCATION

Anticholinergic effects
• Dry mouth
• Blurred vision
• Photophobia
• Urinary hesitancy or retention
• Constipation
• Tachycardia
	• Suggest the following strategies to decrease anticholinergic effects:
	  ○ Chewing sugarless gum
	  ○ Sipping on water
	  ○ Avoiding hazardous activities
	  ○ Wearing sunglasses when outdoors
	  ○ Eating foods high in fiber
	  ○ Participating in regular exercise
	  ○ Maintaining fluid intake of 2 to 3 L/day from beverages and food sources
	  ○ Voiding just before taking medication

Orthostatic hypotension	• The client should develop tolerance in 2 to 3 months. • Monitor the client's blood pressure and heart rate for orthostatic changes. Hold medication until the provider is notified of significant changes. • Instruct clients about the signs of postural hypotension (lightheadedness, dizziness). If these occur, advise the client to sit or lie down. Orthostatic hypotension can be minimized by getting up or changing positions slowly.
Sedation	• Inform the client that effects should diminish within a few weeks. • Instruct the client to take the medication at bedtime to avoid daytime sleepiness. • Advise the client not to drive until sedation has subsided.
Neuroendocrine effects • Gynecomastia • Galactorrhea • Menstrual irregularities	• Advise the client to observe for these manifestations and to notify the provider if they occur.
Seizures • Greatest risk in those clients who have an existing seizure disorder	• Advise the client to report seizure activity to the provider. • An increase in antiseizure medication may be necessary.
Sexual dysfunction, which is common in both males and females	• Advise the client of possible side effects. • Encourage that the client report side effects to the provider. • The client may need dosage lowered or be switched to a high-potency agent.

SIDE/ADVERSE EFFECTS	NURSING INTERVENTIONS/CLIENT EDUCATION
Skin effects • Photosensitivity that can result in severe sunburn • Contact dermatitis from handling medications	• Advise clients to avoid excessive exposure to sunlight, to use sunscreen, and to wear protective clothing. • Advise the client to avoid direct contact with the medication.
Agranulocytosis	• Advise the client to observe for signs of infection (fever, sore throat), and to notify the provider if these occur. • If signs of infection appear, obtain the client's baseline WBC. Medication should be discontinued if laboratory test indicates the presence of infection.
Severe dysrhythmias, which are associated with some of the conventional antipsychotic agents	• Obtain the client's baseline ECG and potassium level prior to treatment, and periodically throughout the treatment period. • Avoid concurrent use with other medications that prolong QT interval.

Ⓢ Contraindications/Precautions

- These medications are contraindicated in clients who are in a coma, or those who have severe depression, Parkinson's disease, prolactin-dependent cancer of the breast, and severe hypotension.

Ⓖ
- Use of conventional antipsychotic medications is contraindicated in older adult clients with dementia.

- Use cautiously in clients with glaucoma, paralytic ileus, prostate enlargement, heart disorders, liver or kidney disease, and seizure disorders.

Medication/Food Interactions

MEDICATION/FOOD INTERACTIONS	NURSING INTERVENTIONS/CLIENT EDUCATION
Anticholinergic agents – concurrent use with other anticholinergic medications will increase effects.	• Advise the client to avoid OTC medications that contain anticholinergic agents, such as sleep aids.
CNS depressants – additive CNS depressant effects with concurrent use of alcohol, opioids, and antihistamines	• Advise the client to avoid alcohol and other medications that cause CNS depression. • Advise the client to avoid hazardous activities, such as driving.
Levodopa – by activating dopamine receptors, levodopa counteracts effects of antipsychotic agents.	• Advise the client to avoid concurrent use of levodopa and other direct dopamine receptor agonists.

Nursing Administration

- Assess client to differentiate between EPS and worsening of a psychotic disorder.

- Administer anticholinergics, beta-blockers, and benzodiazepines to control early EPS. If symptoms are intolerable, a client can be switched to a low-potency or an atypical antipsychotic agent.

- Advise clients that antipsychotic medications do not cause addiction.

- Advise clients to take medication as prescribed and to take it on a regular schedule.

- Advise clients that some therapeutic effects may be noticeable within a few days, but significant improvement may take 2 to 4 weeks, and possibly several months for full effects.

- Consider depot preparations, administered IM once every 2 to 4 weeks, for clients with difficulty maintaining medication regimen. Inform the client that lower doses can be used with depot preparations, which will decrease the risk of adverse effects and the development of tardive dyskinesia.

- Begin administration with twice daily dosing, but switch to daily dosing at bedtime to decrease daytime drowsiness and promote sleep.

MEDICATION CLASSIFICATION: ANTIPSYCHOTICS-ATYPICAL

- Select Prototype Medication: Risperidone (Risperdal)

- Other Medications

  - Olanzapine (Zyprexa)

  - Quetiapine (Seroquel)

  - Aripiprazole (Abilify)

  - Ziprasidone (Geodon)

  - Clozapine (Clozaril)

Purpose

- Expected Pharmacological Action

  - These antipsychotic agents work mainly by blocking serotonin, and to a lesser degree, dopamine receptors. These medications also block receptors for norepinephrine, histamine, and acetylcholine.

- Therapeutic Uses

  - Negative and positive symptoms of schizophrenia

  - Psychosis induced by levodopa therapy

  - Relief of psychotic symptoms in other disorders, such as bipolar disorder

Complications

SIDE/ADVERSE EFFECTS	NURSING INTERVENTIONS/CLIENT EDUCATION
New onset of diabetes mellitus or loss of glucose control in clients with diabetes	• Obtain the client's baseline fasting blood glucose, and monitor the value periodically throughout treatment. • Instruct the client to report signs and symptoms, such as increased thirst, urination, and appetite, to the provider.
Weight gain	• Advise the client to follow a healthy, low-caloric diet, engage in regular exercise, and monitor weight gain.
Hypercholesterolemia with increased risk for hypertension and other cardiovascular disease	• Monitor the client's cholesterol, triglycerides, and blood glucose if weight gain is > 14 kg (30 lb).
Orthostatic hypotension	• Monitor the client's blood pressure and heart rate for orthostatic changes. • Hold medication while notifying the provider of significant changes.
Anticholinergic effects, such as urinary hesitancy or retention, dry mouth	• Monitor for these adverse effects, and report their occurrence to the provider. • Encourage the client to use measures to relieve dry mouth, such as sipping fluids throughout the day.
Symptoms of agitation, dizziness, sedation, and sleep disruption	• Monitor for these adverse effects, and report their occurrence to the provider. • Administer an alternative medication if prescribed.
May cause mild EPS, such as tremor	• Monitor for and teach clients to recognize EPS. • Use AIMS test to screen for EPS.

(S) **Contraindications/Precautions**

- Risperidone

    o Risperidone is a pregnancy risk category C medication.

    o These medications should not be used for dementia-related psychosis. Use of these medications may cause death related to cerebrovascular accident or infection.

    o Clients should avoid the concurrent use of alcohol.

    o Use cautiously in clients with cardiovascular or cerebrovascular disease, seizures, or diabetes mellitus. Clients with diabetes mellitus should have a baseline fasting blood sugar, and blood glucose should be monitored carefully.

- Other Atypical Antipsychotic Agents

MEDICATION	FORMULATIONS	COMMENTS

Olanzapine (Zyprexa)	• Tablets
	• Oral solution
	• Short-acting injectable
		• Low risk of EPS
		• High risk of diabetes, weight gain, and dyslipidemia
		• Other adverse effects include:
		  ○ Sedation
		  ○ Orthostatic hypotension
		  ○ Anticholinergic effects

Quetiapine (Seroquel)	Tablets	• Low risk of EPS
		• Moderate risk of diabetes, weight gain, and dyslipidemia
		• Other adverse effects include:
		  ○ Cataracts
		  ○ Sedation
		  ○ Orthostatic hypotension
		  ○ Anticholinergic effects

Aripiprazole (Abilify)	• Tablets
	• Oral solution
		• Low or no risk of EPS
		• Low or no risk of diabetes, weight gain, dyslipidemia, orthostatic hypotension, and anticholinergic effects
		• Adverse effects include:
		  ○ Sedation
		  ○ Headache
		  ○ Anxiety
		  ○ Insomnia
		  ○ Gastrointestinal upset

MEDICATION	FORMULATIONS	COMMENTS

Ziprasidone (Geodon) – This medication affects both dopamine and serotonin, so it can be used for clients with concurrent depression.	• Capsules
	• Short-acting injectable
		• Low risk of EPS
		• Low risk of diabetes, weight gain, and dyslipidemia
		• Other adverse effects include:
		  ○ Sedation
		  ○ Orthostatic hypotension
		  ○ Anticholinergic effects
		  ○ ECT changes and QT prolongation that may lead to *torsades de pointes*

Clozapine (Clozaril) – The first atypical antipsychotic developed, it is no longer considered a first-line medication for schizophrenia due to its adverse effects.	Tablets	• Low risk of EPS
		• High risk of weight gain, diabetes, and dyslipidemia
		• Risk for fatal agranulocytosis
		  ○ Baseline and weekly monitoring of WBC recommended
		  ○ Notification of the provider of signs of infection (fever, sore throat, mouth lesions) necessary
		• Other adverse effects include:
		  ○ Sedation
		  ○ Orthostatic hypotension
		  ○ Anticholinergic effects

Medication/Food Interactions

MEDICATION/FOOD INTERACTIONS	NURSING INTERVENTIONS/CLIENT EDUCATION
Immunosuppressive medications, such as anticancer medications, can further suppress immune function.	• Avoid use in clients who are taking clozapine.
Additive CNS depressant effects can occur with concurrent use of alcohol, opioids, antihistamines, and other CNS depressants.	• Advise the client to avoid alcohol and other medications that cause CNS depression. • Advise clients to avoid hazardous activities, such as driving.

MEDICATION/FOOD INTERACTIONS	NURSING INTERVENTIONS/CLIENT EDUCATION
Levodopa – by activating dopamine receptors, levodopa counteracts the effects of antipsychotic agents.	• Avoid concurrent use of levodopa and other direct dopamine receptor agonists.
Tricyclic antidepressants, amiodarone (Cordarone), and clarithromycin (Biaxin) prolong QT intervals, thereby increasing the risk of cardiac dysrhythmias.	• Avoid concurrent use with ziprasidone.
Barbiturates and phenytoin (Dilantin) stimulate hepatic drug-metabolizing enzymes, thereby decreasing drug levels of aripiprazole, quetiapine, and ziprasidone.	• Monitor medication effectiveness.
Fluconazole (Diflucan) inhibits hepatic drug-metabolizing enzymes, thereby increasing drug levels of aripiprazole, quetiapine, and ziprasidone.	• Monitor medication effectiveness.

Nursing Administration

- Administer by oral or IM route. Risperidone is also available as a depot injection administered IM once every 2 weeks. This method of administration is a good option for clients who have difficulty adhering to a medication schedule. Therapeutic effect occurs 4 to 6 weeks after first depot injection.

- Advise clients that low doses of medication are given initially and are then gradually increased.

- Use oral disintegrating tablets for clients who may attempt to "cheek" or "pocket" tablets, or for those who have difficulty swallowing them.

Nursing Evaluation of Medication Effectiveness

- Depending on therapeutic intent, effectiveness may be evidenced by:

  ○ Improvement of symptoms (prevention of acute psychotic symptoms, absence of hallucinations, delusions, anxiety, hostility)

  ○ Improvement in ability to perform ADLs

  ○ Improvement in ability to interact socially with peers

  ○ Improvement of sleeping and eating habits

CHAPTER 22: MEDICATIONS FOR PSYCHOSES

(A) Application Exercises

Scenario: A 24-year-old client with paranoid schizophrenia has been treated successfully on an outpatient basis for the past 3 years. Because his condition is deteriorating, he has been admitted to an acute care mental health facility. The client is very suspicious of the nursing staff, and he has auditory hallucinations in which a voice tells him to "hurt those evil people before they hurt you." He also has pressured speech and speaks mostly using clang associations (meaningless rhymes). His appearance indicates a lack of grooming and hygiene. His behavior is usually aggressive toward others, but his face shows no emotion, even though he sounds angry. The provider has prescribed risperidone (Risperdal) oral disintegrating tablets, which the client receives once daily.

1. Which of the client's symptoms indicates a need for an atypical antipsychotic agent rather than a conventional antipsychotic medication?

2. Why is this client receiving tablets that disintegrate on the tongue with or without water versus regular tablets that are swallowed?

3. Which of the following manifestations of schizophrenia are effectively treated by conventional antipsychotics? (Select all that apply.)

    _____ Auditory hallucinations

    _____ Withdrawal from social situations

    _____ Delusions of grandeur

    _____ Loose associations

    _____ Lack of energy

    _____ Lack of motivation to initiate tasks, such as grooming

    _____ Pressured speech

4. Extrapyramidal side effects (EPS) resulting from conventional antipsychotic medications include which of the following? (Select all that apply.)

    _____ Cardiac dysrhythmias

    _____ Parkinson-like symptoms

    _____ Involuntary pelvic and hip movements

    _____ GI pain with nausea, vomiting, and diarrhea

    _____ Muscle spasm in the neck

    _____ Restlessness, jitteriness

    _____ Dehydration caused by polyuria

5. Which of the following client statements indicates understanding of the nurse's teaching regarding antipsychotic medications?

    A. "I will be able to stop taking the drug as soon as I feel better."

    B. "If I feel sleepy I will stop taking the drug and call my provider."

    C. "My symptoms can come back if I don't take the medication exactly as ordered."

    D. "These drugs are highly addictive and must be withdrawn slowly."

6. A client who has been taking an antipsychotic medication for several years begins to exhibit lip smacking, tongue protrusion, and facial grimaces. Which of the following should the nurse suspect?

    A. Parkinsonism

    B. Tardive dyskinesia

    C. Antiadrenergic effects

    D. Anticholinergic effects

CHAPTER 22: MEDICATIONS FOR PSYCHOSES

(A) Application Exercises Answer Key

Scenario: A 24-year-old client with paranoid schizophrenia has been treated successfully on an outpatient basis for the past 3 years. Because his condition is deteriorating, he has been admitted to an acute care mental health facility. The client is very suspicious of the nursing staff, and he has auditory hallucinations in which a voice tells him to "hurt those evil people before they hurt you." He also has pressured speech and speaks mostly using clang associations (meaningless rhymes). His appearance indicates a lack of grooming and hygiene. His behavior is usually aggressive toward others, but his face shows no emotion, even though he sounds angry. The provider has prescribed risperidone (Risperdal) oral disintegrating tablets, which the client receives once daily.

1. Which of the client's symptoms indicates a need for an atypical antipsychotic agent rather than a conventional antipsychotic medication?

> **The negative symptoms of schizophrenia are more readily treated by atypical antipsychotics, such as risperidone, than by conventional antipsychotics, such as chlorpromazine (Thorazine). Negative symptoms for this client include his lack of grooming and hygiene, and his flat affect (no facial emotion). The other symptoms mentioned are positive symptoms of psychosis.**

 NCLEX® Connection: Pharmacological and Parenteral Therapies, Expected Actions/ Outcomes

2. Why is this client receiving tablets that disintegrate on the tongue with or without water versus regular tablets that are swallowed?

> **A client who is suspicious of others and who is so ill that he is unable to behave rationally is at high risk for nonadherence to his treatment regimen. The orally disintegrating tablets dissolve easily in the oral cavity and should help prevent him from "cheeking" his medication and later disposing of it.**

 NCLEX® Connection: Pharmacological and Parenteral Therapies, Medication Administration

3. Which of the following manifestations of schizophrenia are effectively treated by conventional antipsychotics? (Select all that apply.)

  __X__   **Auditory hallucinations**

  _____   Withdrawal from social situations

  __X__   **Delusions of grandeur**

  __X__   **Loose associations**

  _____   Lack of energy

  _____   Lack of motivation to initiate tasks, such as grooming

  __X__   **Pressured speech**

Auditory hallucinations, delusions of grandeur, loose associations, and pressured speech are all positive symptoms of schizophrenia that can be successfully treated with conventional antipsychotics, such as chlorpromazine. Withdrawal from social situations, lack of energy, and no motivation to initiate tasks are examples of negative symptoms. The newer atypical antipsychotics are more effective in treating both positive and negative symptoms.

 NCLEX® Connection: Pharmacological and Parenteral Therapies, Expected Actions/ Outcomes

4. Extrapyramidal side effects (EPS) resulting from conventional antipsychotic medications include which of the following? (Select all that apply.)

  _____   Cardiac dysrhythmias

  __X__   **Parkinson-like symptoms**

  __X__   **Involuntary pelvic and hip movements**

  _____   GI pain with nausea, vomiting, and diarrhea

  __X__   **Muscle spasm in the neck**

  __X__   **Restlessness, jitteriness**

  _____   Dehydration caused by polyuria

EPS involve uncontrollable motor symptoms caused by dopamine receptor blockade and include Parkinson-like symptoms, involuntary pelvic and hip movements, muscle spasm in the neck, restlessness, and jitteriness. Cardiac dysrhythmias, GI pain with nausea, vomiting and diarrhea, and dehydration caused by polyuria are not effects on the extrapyramidal motor system.

 NCLEX® Connection: Pharmacological and Parenteral Therapies, Adverse Effects/ Contraindications/Side Effects/Interactions

5. Which of the following client statements indicates understanding of the nurse's teaching regarding antipsychotic medications?

    A. "I will be able to stop taking the drug as soon as I feel better."

    B. "If I feel sleepy I will stop taking the drug and call my provider."

    C. "My symptoms can come back if I don't take the medication exactly as ordered."

    D. "These drugs are highly addictive and must be withdrawn slowly."

Antipsychotic medications should be taken as ordered to prevent return of psychotic symptoms. Antipsychotic medications are usually taken over a long period of time to prevent symptoms of psychosis. Drowsiness is a common adverse effect of some of the antipsychotic medications; however, stopping the medication if the client feels sleepy is not appropriate. The client should be advised to take the medication at bedtime. Antipsychotic medications are not considered addictive and do not cause tolerance in clients who take them.

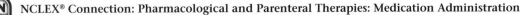 NCLEX® Connection: Pharmacological and Parenteral Therapies: Medication Administration

6. A client who has been taking an antipsychotic medication for several years begins to exhibit lip smacking, tongue protrusion, and facial grimaces. Which of the following should the nurse suspect?

    A. Parkinsonism

    B. Tardive dyskinesia

    C. Antiadrenergic effects

    D. Anticholinergic effects

Tardive dyskinesia includes abnormal movements of the lips, tongue, face, and neck. These symptoms are not characteristic of parkinsonism, antiadrenergic effects, or anticholinergic effects.

NCLEX® Connection: Pharmacological and Parenteral Therapies, Adverse Effects/ Contraindications/Side Effects/Interactions

UNIT 4	PSYCHOPHARMACOLOGICAL THERAPIES
Chapter 23	Medications for Children and Adolescents With Mental Health Issues

Overview

- Various medications may be used to manage behavioral disorders in children and adolescents. Parents should understand that pharmacological management should be accompanied by behavioral modification techniques.

- Medications include selective serotonin reuptake inhibitors, tricyclic antidepressants, antipsychotics, nonbarbiturate anxiolytics, CNS stimulants, and norepinephrine selective reuptake inhibitors.

MEDICATION CLASSIFICATION: SELECTIVE SEROTONIN REUPTAKE INHIBITORS (SSRIs)

- Select Prototype Medication: Fluoxetine (Prozac)

- Other Medications

  o Citalopram (Celexa)

  o Escitalopram oxalate (Lexapro)

  o Paroxetine (Paxil)

  o Sertraline (Zoloft)

Purpose

- Expected Pharmacological Action

  o SSRIs selectively block reuptake of the monoamine neurotransmitter serotonin in the synaptic space, thereby intensifying the effects of the serotonin.

- Therapeutic Uses

  o Major depression

  o Bulimia nervosa

  o Panic, school phobia, separation anxiety disorder

  o Posttraumatic stress disorder (PTSD)

  o Obsessive compulsive disorder (OCD)

  o Attention Deficit Hyperactivity Disorder ADHD

Complications

SIDE/ADVERSE EFFECTS	NURSING INTERVENTIONS/CLIENT EDUCATION
CNS stimulation (inability to sleep, agitation, anxiety)	• Advise the client to notify provider. Dose may need to be lowered. • Advise the client to take dose in the morning. • Advise the client to avoid chocolate and caffeinated beverages. • Teach relaxation techniques to promote sleep.
Weight loss early in therapy may be followed by weight gain with long-term treatment.	• Monitor the client's weight. • Encourage the client to participate in regular exercise and to follow a healthy, well-balanced diet. • Caloric restriction may be warranted.
Serotonin syndrome may begin 2 to 72 hr after starting treatment, and it may be lethal. Manifestations include: • Mental confusion, difficulty concentrating • Agitation • Anxiety • Hallucinations • Incoordination, hyperreflexia • Tremors • Diaphoresis • Fever	• Advise the client to observe for symptoms. If symptoms occur, instruct the client to notify the provider and stop the medication.
Withdrawal syndrome (headache, nausea, visual disturbances, anxiety)	• Instruct the client to taper the dose gradually.
Rash	• Advise the client that a rash can be treated with an antihistamine or the cessation of the medication.
Sleepiness, faintness, lightheadedness	• Advise the client that these side effects are not common, but they can occur. • Instruct the client to avoid driving if these side effects occur.
GI bleeding	• Use caution in clients with a history of GI bleed and ulcers, and in clients taking other medications that affect blood coagulation.

SIDE/ADVERSE EFFECTS	NURSING INTERVENTIONS/CLIENT EDUCATION
Bruxism	• Instruct the client to report this to the provider. • Advise the client to use a mouth guard, and that changing to a different classification of antidepressants, or adding a low dose of buspirone (BuSpar) may be indicated.

 Contraindications/Precautions

- SSRIs are contraindicated in clients taking monoamine oxidase inhibitors (MAOIs) and tricyclic antidepressants (TCAs).

- Use cautiously in clients with liver and renal dysfunction, cardiac disease, seizure disorders, diabetes, ulcers, and a history of GI bleeding.

Medication/Food Interactions

MEDICATION/FOOD INTERACTIONS	NURSING INTERVENTIONS/CLIENT EDUCATION
MAOIs – concurrent use increases the risk of serotonin syndrome.	• MAOIs should be discontinued 14 days prior to starting an SSRI. If already taking fluoxetine, a client should wait 5 weeks before starting an MAOI. • Advise the client to avoid concurrent use with tricyclic antidepressants.
Warfarin (Coumadin) – fluoxetine can displace warfarin from bound protein and result in increased warfarin levels.	• Monitor the client's prothrombin time and INR levels. • Assess the client for signs of bleeding. • A dosage adjustment may be required.
Tricyclic antidepressants and lithium – fluoxetine can increase the levels of these medications.	• Advise the client to avoid concurrent use.
NSAIDs and anticoagulants – fluoxetine suppresses platelet aggregation and thus increases the risk of bleeding when used concurrently with these medications.	• Advise the client to monitor for signs of bleeding (bruising, hematuria) and to notify the provider if they occur.

Nursing Administration

- Assess for the use of alcohol and other CNS depressants, especially with adolescents.

- Medications may be taken with food. Sleep disturbances may be minimized by taking the medication in the morning.

- Instruct the client to take the medication on a daily basis to establish therapeutic plasma levels.

- Suggest weekly dosing for clients with difficulty maintaining compliance.

- Assist the client with medication regimen compliance by informing the client that optimal therapeutic effects may not be experienced for 1 to 3 weeks.

- Instruct the client to continue therapy after improvement in symptoms. Sudden discontinuation of medication can result in relapse.

Nursing Evaluation of Medication Effectiveness

- Effectiveness for clients diagnosed with depression may be evidenced by:

    o   Verbalization of improvement in mood.

    o   Improved sleeping and eating habits

    o   Increased interaction with peers

- Effectiveness for clients diagnosed with ADHD may be evidenced by:

    ▪   Less hyperactivity

    ▪   Greater ability to pay attention

MEDICATION CLASSIFICATION: TRICYCLIC ANTIDEPRESSANTS (TCAs)

- Select Prototype Medication: Amitriptyline (Elavil)

- Other Medications:

    o   Imipramine (Tofranil)

    o   Clomipramine (Anafranil)

    o   Nortriptyline (Aventyl)

Purpose

- Expected Pharmacological Action

    o   These medications block reuptake of the monoamine neurotransmitters norepinephrine and serotonin in the synaptic space, thereby intensifying their effects.

- Therapeutic Uses

    o   Depression

    o   Depressive episodes of bipolar disorders

    o   Autistic disorder

    o   ADHD in children and adults

    o   Panic, school phobia, separation anxiety disorder

    o   PTSD

    o   OCD

Complications

SIDE/ADVERSE EFFECTS	NURSING INTERVENTIONS/CLIENT EDUCATION
Orthostatic hypotension	• Monitor the client's blood pressure with first dose. • If orthostatic hypotension occurs, instruct the client to change positions slowly.

Anticholinergic effects:
• Dry mouth
• Blurred vision
• Photophobia
• Urinary hesitancy or retention
• Constipation
• Tachycardia
	• Instruct the client regarding ways to minimize anticholinergic effects. These include:
	  ○ Chewing sugarless gum
	  ○ Sipping water
	  ○ Avoiding hazardous activities
	  ○ Wearing sunglasses when outdoors
	  ○ Eating foods high in fiber
	  ○ Participating in regular exercise
	  ○ Increasing fluid intake to at least 2 to 3 L/day from beverages and other food sources
	  ○ Voiding just before taking the medication
	• Advise the client to notify the provider if symptoms become intolerable.

Weight gain	• Monitor the client's weight. • Encourage the client to participate in regular exercise and to follow a healthy, low-calorie diet.
Sedation	• Advise the client that side effects should diminish over time • Advise the client to avoid hazardous activities, such as driving if sedation is excessive. • Advise the client to take the medication at bedtime to minimize daytime sleepiness and to promote sleep.
Toxicity resulting in cholinergic blockade and cardiac toxicity evidenced by dysrhythmias, mental confusion, and agitation followed by seizures and coma	• Give a client who is acutely ill a 1-week supply of medication. • Obtain the client's baseline ECG. • Monitor the client's vital signs frequently. • Monitor the client for signs of toxicity. • Notify the provider if signs of toxicity occur.
Decreased seizure threshold	• Monitor clients with seizure disorders.
Excessive sweating	• Inform the client of this side effect, and assist with frequent linen changes.

(S) Contraindications/Precautions

- Use cautiously in clients with seizure disorders; diabetes; liver, kidney and respiratory disorders; and hyperthyroidism.

Medication/Food Interactions

MEDICATION/FOOD INTERACTIONS	NURSING INTERVENTIONS/CLIENT EDUCATION
MAOIs – concurrent use causes hypertension.	Do not administer concurrently with MAOIs.
Antihistamines and other anticholinergic agents – concurrent use may cause additive anticholinergic effects.	Do not administer concurrently with antihistamines.
Epinephrine and dopamine (direct-acting sympathomimetics) – concurrent use may increase hypertensive effect.	Do not administer these medications concurrently with TCAs.
Alcohol, benzodiazepines, opioids, and antihistamines – concurrent use may cause additive CNS depression.	Advise the client to avoid other CNS depressants while taking a TCA.

Nursing Administration

- Instruct the client to take this medication as prescribed on a daily basis to establish therapeutic plasma levels.

- Assist with the client's medication regimen adherence by informing the client that therapeutic effects may not be experienced for 1 to 3 weeks. Full therapeutic effects may not be experienced for 2 to 3 months.

- Instruct the client to continue therapy after improvement in symptoms. Sudden discontinuation of the medication can result in relapse.

(S) - Give only a 1-week supply of medication for a client who is acutely ill, and then only give a 1-month supply of medication at a time.

Nursing Evaluation of Medication Effectiveness

- Effectiveness for clients diagnosed with depression may be evidenced by:

  o Verbalization of improvement in mood.

  o Improved sleeping and eating habits

  o Increased interaction with peers

- Effectiveness for clients diagnosed with autistic disorder may be evidenced by:

  o Decreased anger

  o Decreased compulsive behavior

- Effectiveness for clients diagnosed with ADHD may be evidenced by:

  ○ Decreased hyperactivity

  ○ Greater ability to pay attention

MEDICATION CLASSIFICATION: ATYPICAL ANXIOLYTIC: NONBARBITURATE ANXIOLYTIC

- Select Prototype Medication: Buspirone (BuSpar)

Purpose

- Expected Pharmacological Action

  ○ The exact antianxiety mechanism of this medication is unknown. This medication does bind to serotonin and dopamine receptors. There is no potential for abuse, and use of buspirone does not result in sedation.

- Therapeutic Uses

  ○ Panic disorder, OCD, social anxiety disorder, and PTSD

Complications

SIDE/ADVERSE EFFECTS	NURSING INTERVENTIONS/CLIENT EDUCATION
CNS effects such as dizziness, nausea, headache, agitation	This medication does not interfere with activities, because it does not cause sedation.

 Contraindications/Precautions

- Buspirone is contraindicated for concurrent use with MAOIs, or for 14 days after MAOIs are discontinued. Hypertensive crisis may result.

Medication/Food interactions

MEDICATION/FOOD INTERACTIONS	NURSING INTERVENTIONS/CLIENT EDUCATION
Erythromycin, ketoconazole, and grapefruit juice increase the effect of buspirone.	• Take a complete medication history. • Advise the client to avoid drinking grapefruit juice.

Nursing Administration

- Advise the client to take the medication with meals to prevent gastric irritation.

- Advise the client that effects do not occur rapidly and may take a week before therapeutic benefits are felt, and several weeks longer before the full therapeutic benefit is felt.

Nursing Evaluation of Medication Effectiveness

- Effectiveness for clients diagnosed with depression may be evidenced by:

    o Verbalization of improvement in mood.

    o Improved sleeping and eating habits

    o Increased interaction with peers

- Effectiveness for clients diagnosed with anxiety disorders may be evidenced by:

    o Decrease in anxiety symptoms

    o Improvement in functioning

MEDICATION CLASSIFICATION: CNS STIMULANTS

MEDICATION	SHORT ACTING	INTERMEDIATE ACTING	LONG ACTING
Methylphenidate	Ritalin, Methylin	Ritalin SR, Methylin ER	Ritalin LA, Concerta, Daytrana (transdermal)
Dexmethylphenidate	Focalin		
Dextroamphetamine	Dexedrine		Dexedrine Spansules
Amphetamine Mixture	Adderall		Adderall-XR

Purpose

- Expected Pharmacological Action

    o These medications raise the levels of norepinephrine, serotonin, and dopamine into the central nervous system.

- Therapeutic Uses

    o ADHD in children and adults

    o Conduct disorder

Complications

SIDE/ADVERSE EFFECTS	NURSING INTERVENTIONS/CLIENT EDUCATION
CNS stimulation (insomnia, restlessness)	• Advise the client to observe for symptoms, and if symptoms occur, instruct the client to notify the provider. • Decrease dosage as prescribed. • Administer the last dose of the day before 4 p.m.

SIDE/ADVERSE EFFECTS	NURSING INTERVENTIONS/CLIENT EDUCATION
Weight loss	• Monitor the client's weight and compare to baseline height and weight. • Administer medication right before or after meals. • Encourage children to eat at regular meal times and to avoid unhealthy foods choices.
Cardiovascular effects (dysrhythmias, chest pain, high blood pressure) – may increase the risk of sudden death in clients with heart abnormalities	• Monitor the client's vital signs and ECG. • Advise clients to observe for symptoms and to notify the provider if they occur.
Development of psychotic symptoms, such as hallucinations, paranoia	• Instruct the client to report symptoms immediately and discontinue the medication.
Withdrawal reaction	• Advise the client to avoid abrupt cessation of the medication, as it could lead to depression and severe fatigue.
Hypersensitivity skin reaction to transdermal methylphenidate – hives, papules	• Advise the client to remove the patch and notify the provider.

 Contraindications/Precautions

- Contraindicated in clients with a history of drug abuse, cardiovascular disorders, severe anxiety, and psychosis.

Medication/Food Interactions

MEDICATION/FOOD INTERACTIONS	NURSING INTERVENTIONS/CLIENT EDUCATION
MAOIs – concurrent use may cause hypertensive crisis.	• Avoid concurrent use.
Caffeine – concurrent use may cause an increase in CNS stimulant effects.	• Instruct the client to avoid foods and beverages that contain caffeine.
Phenytoin (Dilantin), warfarin (Coumadin), and phenobarbital – methylphenidate inhibits metabolism of these medications leading to increased serum levels.	• Monitor the client for adverse effects (CNS depression, signs of bleeding). • These medications should be used cautiously together.

MEDICATION/FOOD INTERACTIONS	NURSING INTERVENTIONS/CLIENT EDUCATION
OTC cold and decongestant medications – concurrent use may lead to increased CNS stimulation.	• Instruct the client to avoid the use of these OTC medications.

Nursing Administration

- Advise clients to swallow sustained-release tablets whole and to not chew or crush them.

- Teach the client the importance of administering the medication on a regular schedule.

- Teach clients who use transdermal medication (Daytrana) to place the patch on one hip daily in the morning, and leave it in place no longer than 9 hr. Alternate hips daily.

- Instruct parents and clients that ADHD is not cured by the medication and should be managed in conjunction with an overall treatment plan that may include family and cognitive therapy.

- Instruct parents that these medications have special handling procedures controlled by federal law. Handwritten prescriptions are required for medication refills.

- Instruct parents regarding safety and storage of medications.

- Advise parents that these medications have a high potential for abuse.

Nursing Evaluation of Medication Effectiveness

- Depending on therapeutic intent, effectiveness may be evidenced by:

  o Improvement of symptoms of ADHD, such as an increased ability to focus and complete tasks, interact with peers, and manage impulsivity

---

MEDICATION CLASSIFICATION: NOREPINEPHRINE SELECTIVE REUPTAKE INHIBITOR

- Select Prototype Medication Atomoxetine (Strattera)

Purpose

- Expected Pharmacological Action

  o Block reuptake of norepinephrine at synapses in the CNS. Atomoxetine is not a stimulant medication.

- Therapeutic Uses

  o ADHD in children and adults

Complications

SIDE/ADVERSE EFFECTS	NURSING INTERVENTIONS/CLIENT EDUCATION
Usually tolerated well with minimal side effects	
Appetite suppression, weight loss, growth suppression	• Monitor the client's weight and compare to baseline height and weight. • Administer medication right before meals. • Encourage children to eat at regular meal times and avoid unhealthy food choices.
GI effects (nausea, vomiting)	• Advise the client to take the medication with food if GI effects occur.
Suicidal ideation (in children and adolescents)	• Monitor the client for signs of depression. • Advise the client to report changes in mood, excessive sleeping, agitation, irritability.
Hepatotoxicity	• Advise the client to report signs of liver damage, such as flu-like symptoms, yellowing skin, abdominal pain.

(S) Contraindications/Precautions

- Use cautiously in clients with cardiovascular disorders.

Medication/Food Interactions

MEDICATION/FOOD INTERACTIONS	NURSING INTERVENTIONS/CLIENT EDUCATION
MAOIs – concurrent use may cause hypertensive crisis.	• Advise the client to avoid concurrent use.
Paroxetine (Paxil), fluoxetine (Prozac), or quinidine gluconate (Quinidine) – these medications inhibit metabolizing enzymes, thereby increasing levels of amoxetine.	• Instruct the client to watch for and report increased adverse reactions of amoxetine. • Concurrent use may require a reduction in the dosage of atomoxetine.

Nursing Administration

- Note any changes in the client related to dosing and timing of medications.

- Administer the medication in one daily dose in the morning or in two divided doses, morning and afternoon, with or without food.

- Instruct the client that therapeutic effect may take 1 to 3 weeks to fully develop.

Nursing Evaluation of Medication Effectiveness

- Depending on therapeutic intent, effectiveness may be evidenced by:

  o Improvement of the symptoms of ADHD, such as increase in ability to focus and complete tasks, interact with peers, and manage impulsivity.

MEDICATION CLASSIFICATION: ANTIPSYCHOTICS-ATYPICAL

- Select Prototype Medication: Risperidone (Risperdal)

- Other Medications

  o Olanzapine (Zyprexa)

  o Quetiapine (Seroquel)

Purpose

- Expected Pharmacological Action

  o These antipsychotic agents work mainly by blocking serotonin, and to a lesser degree, dopamine receptors. These medications also block receptors for norepinephrine, histamine, and acetylcholine.

- Therapeutic Uses

  o Pervasive development disorders (PDD), including autistic disorder

  o Conduct disorder

  o PTSD

  o Relief of psychotic symptoms

Complications

SIDE/ADVERSE EFFECTS	NURSING INTERVENTIONS/CLIENT EDUCATION
New onset of diabetes or loss of glucose control in clients with diabetes	• Obtain the client's baseline fasting blood glucose, and monitor periodically throughout treatment. • Instruct the client to report signs and symptoms such as increased thirst, urination, and appetite.
Weight gain	• Advise the client to follow a healthy, low-calorie diet, engage in regular exercise, and monitor weight gain.
Hypercholesterolemia with increased risk for hypertension and other cardiovascular disease	• Monitor cholesterol, triglycerides, and blood glucose if weight gain is more than 14 kg (30 lb).

SIDE/ADVERSE EFFECTS	NURSING INTERVENTIONS/CLIENT EDUCATION
Orthostatic hypotension	• Monitor blood pressure with first dose, and instruct the client to change positions slowly if orthostatic hypotension occurs.
Anticholinergic effects (urinary retention or hesitancy, dry mouth)	• Monitor for these adverse effects, and report their occurrence to the provider. • Encourage client to use measures to relieve dry mouth such as sipping fluids throughout the day.
Symptoms of agitation, dizziness, sedation, and sleep disruption	• Monitor for these adverse effects and report their occurrence to the provider. • Administer an alternative medication if prescribed.
Mild extrapyramidal side effects (EPS), such as tremor	• Monitor for and teach clients to recognize EPS. These effects are usually dose related.

Ⓢ Contraindications/Precautions

- Clients should avoid the use of alcohol.

- Use cautiously in clients with cardiovascular disease, seizures, or diabetes. Clients with diabetes should have a baseline fasting blood sugar, and blood glucose should be monitored carefully.

MEDICATION/FOOD INTERACTIONS	NURSING INTERVENTIONS/CLIENT EDUCATION
CNS depressants – additive CNS depression occurs with concurrent use of alcohol, opioids, antihistamines.	• Advise the client to avoid alcohol and other medications that cause CNS depression. • Advise the client to avoid hazardous activities, such as driving.
Levodopa – by activating dopamine receptors, levodopa counteracts the effects of antipsychotic agents.	Avoid concurrent use of levodopa and other direct dopamine receptor agonists is not recommended.
Tricyclic antidepressants, amiodarone (Cordarone), and clarithromycin (Biaxin) prolong QT interval, thereby increasing the risk of cardiac dysrhythmias.	Avoid concurrent use of these medications.
Barbiturates and phenytoin (Dilantin) promote hepatic drug-metabolizing enzymes, thereby decreasing drug levels of quetiapine.	Monitor medication for effectiveness.
Fluconazole (Diflucan) inhibits hepatic drug-metabolizing enzymes, thereby increasing drug levels of aripiprazole, quetiapine, and ziprasidone.	Monitor the client for adverse medication effects.

Nursing Administration

- Administer by oral or IM route.

- Advise clients that low doses of medication are given initially and are then gradually increased.

Nursing Evaluation of Medication Effectiveness

- Effectiveness for clients diagnosed with PPD may be evidenced by:

  ○ Reduction of hyperactivity

  ○ Improvement in mood

- Effectiveness for clients diagnosed with conduct disorder may be evidenced by:

  ○ Decreased aggressiveness

- Effectiveness for clients diagnosed with PTSD may be evidenced by:

  ○ Decreased aggressiveness and reduction of flashbacks

  ○ Improvement of psychotic symptoms (prevention of acute psychotic symptoms, absence of hallucinations, delusions, anxiety, hostility)

  ○ Improvement in ability to perform ADLs

  ○ Improvement in ability to interact socially with peers

  ○ Improvement of sleeping and eating habits

CHAPTER 23: MEDICATIONS FOR CHILDREN AND ADOLESCENTS WITH MENTAL HEALTH ISSUES

 Application Exercises

1. A nurse is teaching a child with a new prescription for paroxetine (Paxil) and his parents about reactions to watch for during the first 3 days of treatment. For which of the following manifestations should the nurse teach the family to discontinue the medication and notify the provider immediately? (Select all that apply.)

_____ Agitation

_____ Fever

_____ Nausea

_____ Headache

_____ Tremors

2. An adolescent client has just begun taking amitriptyline (Elavil) for depression. Which of the following nursing interventions should the nurse teach the client to minimize one of the adverse effects of his medication?

    A. Eat a diet high in fiber.

    B. Check temperature daily.

    C. Take medication first thing in the morning before eating.

    D. Add extra calories to the diet as between-meal snacks.

3. A nurse is providing teaching to an adolescent who is to begin taking buspirone (BuSpar) for an anxiety disorder. Which of the following foods should the nurse instruct the client to avoid?

    A. Chicken

    B. Cheddar cheese

    C. Grapefruit juice

    D. Whole wheat bread

4. A nurse is caring for a school age child who has been prescribed methylphenidate (Daytrana) to treat ADHD. Which of the following should the nurse teach the client and family about this medication?

    A. Apply the patch once daily at bedtime.

    B. Take oral medication once daily in the morning.

    C. Take oral medication early in the morning and again at bedtime.

    D. Apply the patch on awakening and remove at bedtime.

CHAPTER 23: MEDICATIONS FOR CHILDREN AND ADOLESCENTS WITH MENTAL HEALTH ISSUES

 Application Exercises Answer Key

1. A nurse is teaching a child with a new prescription for paroxetine (Paxil) and his parents about reactions to watch for during the first 3 days of treatment. For which of the following manifestations should the nurse teach the family to discontinue the medication and notify the provider immediately? (Select all that apply.)

   __X__   **Agitation**

   __X__   **Fever**

   _____   Nausea

   _____   Headache

   __X__   **Tremors**

    Agitation, fever, and tremors, as well as hyperreflexia and hallucinations are some of the manifestations of serotonin syndrome, which may occur between 2 and 72 hr after beginning treatment with paroxetine and other SSRI medications. The client should discontinue the medication and notify the provider if these symptoms occur. Nausea and headache are signs of abrupt withdrawal from SSRI medications and are not manifestations to watch for during the first 3 days of therapy.

 NCLEX® Connection: Pharmacological and Parenteral Therapies, Adverse Effects/ Contraindications/Side Effects/Interactions

2. An adolescent client has just begun taking amitriptyline (Elavil) for depression. Which of the following nursing interventions should the nurse teach the client to minimize one of the adverse effects of his medication?

    A. Eat a diet high in fiber.

    B. Check temperature daily.

    C. Take medication first thing in the morning before eating.

    D. Add extra calories to the diet as between-meal snacks.

    Eating foods high in fiber will help prevent constipation, an anticholinergic effect that may occur when taking a TCA, such as amitriptyline. Checking the temperature daily while taking a TCA is not necessary. Taking the medication at bedtime rather than in the morning will prevent daytime sleepiness. Following a low-calorie diet rather than adding extra calories will help prevent weight gain, a common adverse effect.

 NCLEX® Connection: Pharmacological and Parenteral Therapies, Adverse Effects/ Contraindications/Side Effects/Interactions

3. A nurse is providing teaching to an adolescent who is to begin taking buspirone (BuSpar) for an anxiety disorder. Which of the following foods should the nurse instruct the client to avoid?

    A. Chicken

    B. Cheddar cheese

    C. Grapefruit juice

    D. Whole wheat bread

    Grapefruit juice can increase the effects of buspirone and should be avoided. There are no contraindications to eating chicken, cheddar cheese, or whole wheat bread.

 NCLEX® Connection: Pharmacological and Parenteral Therapies: Adverse Effects/ Contraindications/Side Effects/Interactions

4. A nurse is caring for a school age child who has been prescribed methylphenidate (Daytrana) to treat ADHD. Which of the following should the nurse teach the client and family about this medication?

    A. Apply the patch once daily at bedtime.

    B. Take oral medication once daily in the morning.

    C. Take oral medication early in the morning and again at bedtime.

    D. Apply the patch on awakening and remove at bedtime.

    A long-acting methylphenidate (Daytrana) is available as a transdermal patch, which should be put on in the morning and removed after no more than 9 hr each day. Concerta is a long-acting formulation of methylphenidate that should be taken once daily in the morning. Short-acting methylphenidate (Ritalin) is taken orally two or three times daily; however, the last dose is taken no later than late afternoon or early evening, so as not to interfere with sleep.

 NCLEX® Connection: Pharmacological and Parenteral Therapies: Expected Actions/ Outcomes

UNIT 4   PSYCHOPHARMACOLOGICAL THERAPIES

Chapter 24   Medications for Substance Abuse

Overview

- Abstinence syndrome occurs when a client abruptly withdraws from a drug on which he is physically dependent.

- Withdrawing from a substance that has the potential to cause abstinence syndrome can cause distressing symptoms that can also be life threatening.

MAJOR DRUGS OF ABUSE	
SUBSTANCE	**WITHDRAWAL SYMPTOMS**
Alcohol	• Symptoms usually start within 4 to 12 hr of the last intake of alcohol, peak after 24 to 48 hr, and then suddenly disappear, unless alcohol withdrawal delirium occurs. • Common symptoms include nausea; vomiting; tremors; restlessness and inability to sleep; depressed mood or irritability; increased heart rate, blood pressure, respiratory rate, and temperature; and tonic-clonic seizures. Illusions are also common. • Alcohol withdrawal delirium may occur 2 to 3 days after cessation of alcohol and may last 2 to 3 days. This is considered a medical emergency. Symptoms include severe disorientation, psychotic symptoms (hallucinations), severe hypertension, cardiac dysrhythmias, and delirium. This type of withdrawal may progress to death.
Opioids, including heroin, as well as prescription medications	• Withdrawal symptoms occur within hours to several days after cessation of drug use. • Common symptoms include agitation, insomnia, flu-like symptoms, rhinorrhea, yawning, sweating, and diarrhea. • Withdrawal symptoms are not life threatening, although suicidal ideation may occur.
Nicotine	• Abstinence syndrome is evidenced by irritability, nervousness, restlessness, insomnia, and difficulty concentrating.

MEDICATIONS TO SUPPORT WITHDRAWAL/ABSTINENCE FROM ALCOHOL

Detoxification

- Benzodiazepines

    o Chlordiazepoxide (Librium)

    o Diazepam (Valium)

    o Lorazepam (Ativan)

INTENDED EFFECTS	NURSING INTERVENTIONS/CLIENT EDUCATION
• Maintenance of the client's vital signs within normal limits • Decrease in the risk of seizures • Decrease in the intensity of symptoms	• Administer around the clock or PRN. • Obtain the client's baseline vital signs. • Monitor the client's vital signs and neurological status on an ongoing basis. • Provide for seizure precautions (padded side rails, suction equipment at bedside).

- Adjunct Medications

    o Carbamazepine (Tegretol)

    o Clonidine (Catapres)

    o Propranolol (Inderal)

INTENDED EFFECTS	NURSING INTERVENTIONS/CLIENT EDUCATION
• Decrease in seizures - carbamazepine • Depression of autonomic response (decrease in blood pressure, heart rate) – clonidine and propranolol • Decrease in craving - propranolol	• Provide for seizure precautions (padded side rails, suction equipment at bedside). • Obtain the client's baseline vital signs and continue to monitor on a regular basis.

Abstinence Maintenance (Following Detoxification)

- Disulfiram (Antabuse)

INTENDED EFFECTS	NURSING INTERVENTIONS/CLIENT EDUCATION
• Disulfiram is a daily oral medication that is a type of aversion (behavioral) therapy. • Disulfiram used concurrently with alcohol will cause acetaldehyde syndrome to occur. ○ Effects include nausea, vomiting, weakness, sweating, palpitations, and hypotension. • Acetaldehyde syndrome can progress to respiratory depression, cardiovascular suppression, seizures, and death.	• Inform the client of the potential dangers of drinking any alcohol. • Advise the client to avoid any products that contain alcohol (cough syrups, aftershave lotion). • Encourage the client to wear a medical alert bracelet. • Encourage the client to participate in a 12-step program. • Advise the client that medication effects, such as the potential for acetaldehyde syndrome with alcohol ingestion, persist for 2 weeks following discontinuation of disulfiram.

- Naltrexone (ReVia)

INTENDED EFFECTS	NURSING INTERVENTIONS/CLIENT EDUCATION
Naltrexone is a pure opioid antagonist that suppresses the craving and pleasurable effects of alcohol (also used for opioid withdrawal).	• Assess the client's history to determine if the client is also dependent on opioids. Use of naltrexone will initiate withdrawal syndrome. • Advise the client to take naltrexone with meals to decrease gastrointestinal distress. • Suggest monthly IM injections for clients who have difficulty adhering to the medication regimen.

- Acamprosate (Campral)

INTENDED EFFECTS	NURSING INTERVENTIONS/CLIENT EDUCATION
Acamprosate decreases unpleasant effects resulting from abstinence (anxiety, restlessness).	• Inform the client that diarrhea may result. • Advise the client to maintain adequate fluid intake and to get adequate rest. • Advise the client to avoid use in pregnancy.

MEDICATIONS TO SUPPORT WITHDRAWAL/ABSTINENCE FROM OPIOIDS

- Methadone (Dolophine) Substitution

INTENDED EFFECTS	NURSING INTERVENTIONS/CLIENT EDUCATION
• Methadone substitution is an oral opioid agonist that replaces the opioid to which the client is addicted. • This will prevent abstinence syndrome from occurring and remove the need for the client to obtain illegal drugs. • Methadone substitution is used for withdrawal and long-term maintenance. • Dependence will be transferred from the illegal opioid to methadone.	• Inform the client that the methadone dose must be slowly tapered during detoxification. • Encourage the client to participate in a 12-step program. • Inform the client that the medication must be administered from an approved treatment center.

- Clonidine (Catapres)

INTENDED EFFECTS	NURSING INTERVENTIONS/CLIENT EDUCATION
• Clonidine assists with withdrawal symptoms related to autonomic hyperactivity (diarrhea, nausea, vomiting). • Clonidine therapy does not reduce the craving for opioids.	• Obtain baseline vital signs. • Advise the client to avoid activities that require mental alertness until symptoms of drowsiness subside. • Encourage the client to chew on gum or hard candy and to sip on small amounts of water or suck on ice chips to treat dry mouth.

- Buprenorphine (Subutex), Buprenorphine Combined with Naloxone (Suboxone)

INTENDED EFFECTS	NURSING INTERVENTIONS/CLIENT EDUCATION
• These medications are agonist-antagonist opioids used for both detoxification and maintenance. • These medications decrease feelings of craving and may be effective in maintaining compliance.	• Inform the client that the medication must be administered from an approved treatment center. • Administer the medications sublingually.

MEDICATIONS TO SUPPORT WITHDRAWAL/ABSTINENCE FROM NICOTINE

- Bupropion (Zyban)

INTENDED EFFECTS	NURSING INTERVENTIONS/CLIENT EDUCATION
Bupropion decreases nicotine craving and symptoms of withdrawal.	<ul><li>To treat dry mouth, encourage the client to chew on gum or hard candy and to sip on small amounts of water or suck on ice chips.</li><li>Advise the client to avoid caffeine and other CNS stimulants to control insomnia.</li></ul>

- Nicotine Replacement Therapy (Nicotine Gum [Nicorette] and Nicotine Patch [Nicotrol])

INTENDED EFFECTS	NURSING INTERVENTIONS/CLIENT EDUCATION
These nicotine replacements are pharmaceutical product substitutes for the nicotine in cigarettes or chewing tobacco.	<ul><li>Use of chewing gum is not recommended for longer than 6 months.</li><li>Advise the client to:<ul><li>Chew gum slowly and intermittently over 30 min.</li><li>Avoid eating or drinking 15 min prior to and while chewing the gum.</li><li>Apply a nicotine patch to an area of clean, dry skin each day.</li><li>Avoid using any nicotine products while wearing the patch.</li><li>Follow product directions for dosage times.</li><li>Remove the patch and notify the provider if a local skin reaction occurs.</li><li>Avoid using any nicotine products while pregnant or breastfeeding.</li><li>Remove the patch prior to an MRI scan.</li></ul></li></ul>

Nursing Evaluation of Medication Effectiveness

- Depending on therapeutic intent, effectiveness may be evidenced by:

    ○ Absence of injury

    ○ Ongoing abstinence from the substance

    ○ Regular attendance at a 12-step program

CHAPTER 24: MEDICATIONS FOR SUBSTANCE ABUSE

 Application Exercises

1. A nurse is caring for a client who is withdrawing from alcohol. Which of the following medications should the nurse expect to administer to prevent the development of seizures?

    A. Carbamazepine (Tegretol)

    B. Methadone (Dolophine)

    C. Propranolol (Inderal)

    D. Clonidine (Catapres)

2. Which of the following medications may be used to manage long-term management of abstinence from alcohol? (Select all that apply.)

    _____ Lorazepam (Ativan)

    _____ Diazepam (Valium)

    _____ Disulfiram (Antabuse)

    _____ Naltrexone (ReVia)

    _____ Acamprosate (Campral)

3. A nurse is providing teaching to a client who is prescribed clonidine (Catapres) to assist with maintenance of abstinence from opioids. For which of the following side effects should the nurse instruct the client to observe?

    A. Diarrhea

    B. Dry mouth

    C. Agitation

    D. Weight loss

4. Match the treatment goal with the appropriate medication.

_____ Alcohol withdrawal	A. Methadone (Dolophine)
_____ Heroin withdrawal	B. Naloxone (Narcan)
_____ Nicotine withdrawal	C. Bupropion (Zyban)
_____ Alcohol abstinence	D. Chlordiazepoxide (Librium)
_____ Morphine overdose	E. Disulfiram (Antabuse)

CHAPTER 24: MEDICATIONS FOR SUBSTANCE ABUSE

 Application Exercises Answer Key

1. A nurse is caring for a client who is withdrawing from alcohol. Which of the following medications should the nurse expect to administer to prevent the development of seizures?

> **A. Carbamazepine (Tegretol)**
>
> B. Methadone (Dolophine)
>
> C. Propranolol (Inderal)
>
> D. Clonidine (Catapres)

> **Carbamazepine is an antiepileptic agent administered to prevent seizures. Methadone is used for opioid withdrawal. Propranolol is administered to decrease craving and control autonomic responses, such as elevated heart rate and blood pressure. Clonidine provides relief for somatic symptoms of withdrawal.**

> **NCLEX® Connection: Pharmacological and Parenteral Therapies, Adverse Effects/ Contraindications/Side Effects/Interactions**

2. Which of the following medications may be used to manage long-term management of abstinence from alcohol? (Select all that apply.)

> _____ Lorazepam (Ativan)
>
> _____ Diazepam (Valium)
>
> **X   Disulfiram (Antabuse)**
>
> **X   Naltrexone (ReVia)**
>
> **X   Acamprosate (Campral)**

> **Disulfiram is administered to assist the client to maintain abstinence from alcohol. If the client drinks alcohol while taking disulfiram, she may experience a mild reaction, such as nausea and vomiting, or a more severe reaction that can lead to respiratory depression and death. Naltrexone is a pure opioid antagonist that suppresses the craving and pleasurable effects of alcohol. Acamprosate decreases unpleasant effects resulting from abstinence (e.g., anxiety, restlessness). Lorazepam and diazepam are both benzodiazepines used short term for detoxification.**

> **NCLEX® Connection: Pharmacological and Parenteral Therapies, Expected Actions/ Outcomes**

3. A nurse is providing teaching to a client who is prescribed clonidine (Catapres) to assist with maintenance of abstinence from opioids. For which of the following side effects should the nurse instruct the client to observe?

    A. Diarrhea

    B. Dry mouth

    C. Agitation

    D. Weight loss

    Dry mouth is a common side effect of clonidine that can be managed by chewing gum or sipping water throughout the day. Clonidine may cause constipation and drowsiness and is used to decrease the autonomic symptoms of diarrhea and agitation. Weight loss is not associated with clonidine use.

(N) NCLEX® Connection: Pharmacological and Parenteral Therapies, Adverse Effects/ Contraindications/Side Effects/Interactions

4. Match the treatment goal with the appropriate medication.

D	Alcohol withdrawal	A. Methadone (Dolophine)
A	Heroin withdrawal	B. Naloxone (Narcan)
C	Nicotine withdrawal	C. Bupropion (Zyban)
E	Alcohol abstinence	D. Chlordiazepoxide (Librium)
B	Morphine overdose	E. Disulfiram (Antabuse)

(N) NCLEX® Connection: Pharmacological and Parenteral Therapies, Expected Actions/ Outcomes

UNIT 5: SPECIAL POPULATIONS

- Care of Those Who Are Dying and/or Grieving
- Mental Health Issues of Children and Adolescents

NCLEX® CONNECTIONS

When reviewing the chapters in this unit, keep in mind the relevant sections of the NCLEX® outline, in particular:

CLIENT NEEDS: PSYCHOSOCIAL INTEGRITY

Relevant topics/tasks include:
- End-of-Life Care
  - Assist the client in resolution of end-of-life issues.
- Grief and Loss
  - Assist the client in coping with suffering, grief, loss, dying, and bereavement.
  - Inform the client of expected reactions to grief and loss.
- Mental Health Concepts
  - Provide care and education for acute and chronic behavioral health issues.
  - Evaluate the client's ability to adhere to the treatment plan.

Overview

- Clients experience loss in many aspects of their lives.

- Grief is the inner emotional response to loss and is exhibited in as many ways as there are individuals.

- Bereavement includes both grief and mourning (the outward display of loss) as an individual deals with the death of a significant individual.

- Palliative, or end-of-life care, is an important aspect of nursing care that attempts to meet the client's physical and psychosocial needs.

- End-of-life issues include decision making in a highly stressful time during which the nurse must consider the desires of the client and the family. Any decisions must be shared with other health care personnel for a smooth transition during this time of stress, grief, and bereavement.

- Advance directives – Legal documents that direct end-of-life issues.

   o   Living wills – Directive documents for medical treatment per a client's wishes.

   o   Durable power of attorney for health care – A document that appoints an individual to make medical decisions when a client is no longer able to do so on his own behalf.

TYPES OF LOSS	
Necessary loss	Part of the cycle of life, anticipated but may still be intensely felt
Actual loss	Any loss of a valued person or item
Perceived loss	Any loss defined by a client that is not be obvious to others
Maturational loss	Losses normally expected due to the developmental processing of life
Situational loss	Unanticipated loss caused by an external event

Theories of Grief

- Kübler-Ross: Five Stages of Grief – Stages may not be experienced in order, and the length of each stage will vary from person to person.

  o Denial – The client has difficulty believing a terminal diagnosis or loss.

  o Anger – The client lashes out at other people or things.

  o Bargaining – The client negotiates for more time or a cure.

  o Depression – The client is saddened over the inability to change the situation.

  o Acceptance – The client accepts what is happening and plans for the future.

- Worden: Four Tasks of Mourning – Completion of all four tasks generally takes about a year, but this may also vary from person to person.

  o Task I – Accepting the inevitability of the loss

  o Task II – Using coping mechanisms to experience the emotional pain of the loss

  o Task III – Changing the environment to accommodate the absence of the deceased

  o Task IV – Readjusting emotional ties to new individuals, and moving thoughts about the deceased to a less prominent place in everyday thoughts

Factors Influencing Loss, Grief, and Coping Ability

- An individual's current stage of development

- Interpersonal relationships and social support network

- Type and significance of the loss

- Culture and ethnicity

- Spiritual and religious beliefs and practices

- Prior experience with loss

- Socioeconomic status

- Dysfunctional grieving risks

  o Being dependent upon the deceased

  o Unexpected death at a young age, through violence, or by a socially unacceptable manner

  o Inadequate coping skills or lack of social support

  o Pre-existing mental health issues, such as depression or substance abuse

Assessment

TYPES OF GRIEF	
Normal grief	• This grief is considered uncomplicated. • Emotions may be negative loss, such as anger, resentment, withdrawal, hopelessness, and guilt but should change to acceptance with time. • Some acceptance should be evident by 6 months after the loss. • Somatic complaints may include chest pain, palpitations, headaches, nausea, changes in sleep patterns, or fatigue.
Anticipatory grief	• This grief implies the "letting go" of an object or person before the loss, as in the case of a terminal illness. • Individuals have the opportunity to grieve before the actual loss.
Dysfunctional grief	• This grief involves difficult progression through the expected stages of the grieving process. • Usually the work of grief is prolonged, the symptoms are more severe, and they may result in depression or exacerbation of a pre-existing disorder. • The client may develop suicidal ideation, intense feelings of guilt, and lowered self-esteem. • Somatic complaints persist for an extended period of time.
Disenfranchised grief	• This grief entails an experienced loss that cannot be publicly shared or is not socially acceptable, such as the loss of a loved one through suicide.

Nursing Interventions

- Facilitate Mourning

  - Grant time for the grieving process.

  - Identify expected grieving behaviors, such as crying, somatic manifestations, anxiety.

  - Use therapeutic communication. Name the emotion that the client is feeling. For example, a nurse may say, "You sound as though you are angry. Anger is a normal feeling for someone who has lost a loved one. Tell me about how you are feeling."

  - Avoid communication that inhibits open expression of feelings, such as offering false reassurance, giving advice, changing the subject, and taking the focus away from the individual who is grieving.

  - Assist the individual to accept the reality of the loss.

  - Support the client's efforts to "move on" in the face of the loss.

  - Encourage the building of new relationships.

  - Provide continuing support; encourage the support of family and friends.

- Assess for signs of ineffective coping, such as refusing to leave her home months after a client's spouse has died.

- Share information about mourning and grieving with the client, who may not realize that feelings, such as anger toward the deceased, are expected.

- Encourage the client who is grieving to attend a bereavement or grief support group.

- Initiate a referral for psychotherapy for a client who is having difficulty resolving grief.

- Provide information on available community resources.

- Ask the client if contacting a spiritual advisor would be acceptable, or encourage the client to do so.

- Participate in debriefing provided by professional grief/mental health counselors.

Client Outcomes

- Client verbalizes needs to the care provider.

- Client progresses through the stages of grief in a timely manner.

PALLIATIVE CARE

Overview

- The nurse serves as an advocate for a client's sense of dignity and self-esteem by providing palliative care at the end of life.

- Palliative care improves the quality of life of clients and their families facing end-of-life issues.

- Palliative care interventions are used primarily when caring for clients who are dying and family members who are grieving.

- Palliative care can be provided by an interdisciplinary team of:

  - Physicians

  - Nurses

  - Social workers

  - Massage therapists

  - Occupational therapists

  - Music/art therapists

  - Touch/energy therapists

- Hospice care is a comprehensive care delivery system for the terminally ill that is usually implemented when a client is not expected to live longer than 6 months. Further medical care aimed toward a cure is discontinued, and the focus becomes symptom relief and maintaining the client's quality of life.

Assessment

CHARACTERISTICS OF DISCOMFORT	SIGNS AND SYMPTOMS OF APPROACHING DEATH
• Pain • Anxiety • Dyspnea • Nausea or vomiting • Dehydration • Diarrhea or constipation • Urinary incontinence • Inability to perform ADLs	• Decreased level of consciousness • Muscle relaxation • Labored breathing (dyspnea, apnea, Cheyne-Stokes respirations) • Mucus collection in large airways • Incontinence of bowel and/or bladder • Occurrence of mottling with poor circulation • Nonreactive pupils • Weak pulse and dropping blood pressure • Cool extremities • Perspiration • Decreased urine output • Inability to swallow

- Determine the client's sources of strength and hope.

- Identify the desires and expectations of the family and client for end-of-life care.

Nursing Interventions

- Promote continuity of care and communication by limiting assigned staff changes.

- Assist the client and family to set priorities for end-of-life care.

- Physical Care

  o Give priority to the control of symptoms.

  o Administer medications that manage pain, air hunger, and anxiety.

  o Perform ongoing assessment to determine effectiveness of treatment and need for modifications of treatment plan, such as lower or higher doses of medications.

  o Manage side effects of medications.

  o Reposition the client to maintain airway and comfort.

  o Maintain integrity of skin and mucous membranes.

  o Provide an environment that promotes dignity and self-esteem.

    ■ Remove products of elimination as soon as possible to maintain a clean and odor-free environment.

    ■ Offer comfortable clothing.

    ■ Provide grooming for hair, nails, and skin

    ■ Encourage family members to bring in comforting possessions to make the client feel at home.

- o   Encourage use of relaxation techniques, such as guided imagery and music.

- o   Promote decision making in food selection, activities, and health care to permit the client as much control as possible.

- o   Encourage the client to perform ADLs if the ability and desire exist.

- Psychosocial Care

   - o   Use an interdisciplinary approach.

   - o   Provide care to the client and the family.

   - o   Use volunteers when appropriate to provide non medical care.

   - o   Use therapeutic communication to develop and maintain a nurse-client relationship.

   - o   Facilitate understanding of information regarding disease progression and treatment choices.

   - o   Facilitate communication between the client, family, and provider.

   - o   Encourage the client to participate in religious practices that bring comfort and strength, if appropriate.

   - o   Assist the client in clarifying personal values to facilitate effective decision making.

   - o   Encourage the client to use coping mechanisms that have worked in the past.

   - o   Be sensitive to comments made in the presence of a client who is unconscious, as hearing is the last of the senses that is lost.

- Prevention of Abandonment and Isolation

   - o   Prevent the fear of dying alone.

      - ■   Make presence known by answering call lights in a timely manner and making frequent contact.

      - ■   Keep the client informed of procedure/assessment times.

      - ■   Allow family members to spend the night.

      - ■   Determine where the client is most comfortable, such as in a room close to the nurses' station.

- Support for the Grieving Family

   - o   Suggest that family members plan visits in a manner that promotes client rest.

   - o   Ensure that the family receives appropriate information as the treatment plan changes.

   - o   Provide privacy so family members have the opportunity to communicate and express feelings among themselves without including the client.

   - o   Determine family members' desire to provide physical care. Provide instruction as necessary.

   - o   Educate the family about physical changes to expect as the client moves closer to death.

Client Outcomes

- The client verbalizes that pain and discomfort are controlled.

- The client rests comfortably and exhibits minimal signs of distress.

- The client participates in care as much as possible.

POSTMORTEM CARE

Overview

- A nurse is responsible for following federal and state laws regarding requests for organ or tissue donation, obtaining permission for autopsy, certification and appropriate documentation of the death, and providing safe postmortem (after-death) care.

- The client's family now becomes the nurse's primary focus.

Nursing Interventions

- Care of the Body

  ○ Provide care with respect and compassion while attending to the desires of the client and family per their cultural, religious, and social practices.

  ○ Recognize that the provider certifies the client's death by pronouncing time and documenting therapies used, and actions taken prior to the death.

  ○ Preparing the body for viewing includes:

    ▪ Maintaining privacy

    ▪ Shaving facial hair if applicable and/or desired by the family

    ▪ Removing all tubes and soiled linens, unless organs are to be donated or this is a coroner's case

    ▪ Removing all personal belongings to be given to the family

    ▪ Cleansing and positioning the body with a pillow under the head, arms outside the sheet and blanket, dentures in place, and eyes closed.

    ▪ Applying fresh linens and a gown

    ▪ Brushing/combing the client's hair, replacing any hair pieces

    ▪ Removing excess equipment and linens from the room

    ▪ Dimming the lights and minimizing noise to provide a calm environment

- o Viewing considerations include:
    - Asking the family if they would like to remain with the body, honoring any decision. This process should not be rushed.
    - Clarifying where the client's personal belongings should go either with the body or to a designated person.
    - Adhering to the same procedures when the deceased is a newborn, while adding the following:
        - □ Swaddling the infant's body in a clean blanket
        - □ Transporting the cradled infant in the nurse's arms or in a special infant carrier.
        - □ Offering mementos of the infant (identification bracelets, footprints, cord clamp, lock of hair, photos).
- o Post viewing
    - Apply identification tags according to the facility's policy.
    - Complete documentation.
    - Remain aware of visitor and staff sensibilities during transport.

- Organ Donation
    - o Recognize that request for tissue and organ donation must be made by specially trained personnel.
    - o Provide support and education to family members as decisions are being made. Use a private area for any family discussions concerning donation.
    - o Be sensitive to cultural and religious influences.
    - o Maintain ventilatory and cardiovascular support for vital organ retrieval.

- Autopsy Considerations
    - o The provider typically approaches the family about performing an autopsy.
    - o The nurse's role is to answer the family's questions and support the family's choices.
    - o Autopsies can be conducted to advance scientific knowledge regarding disease processes, which can lead to the development of new therapies.
    - o The law may require an autopsy to be performed if the death is due to a homicide, an accident, or if the death occurs within 24 hr of hospital admission.
    - o Most facilities require that equipment used during medical intervention, such as tubes, remain in place if an autopsy is planned.

- Cultural/Religious Beliefs

  o Identify cultural/religious beliefs of family members.

  o Be sensitive to these practices when providing postmortem care.

- Documentation and completion of forms following federal and state laws typically includes:

  o Person pronouncing the death and at what time

  o Consideration of and preparation for organ donation

  o Disposition of personal articles

  o Names of people notified and any decisions made

  o Location of identification tags

  o Time the body left the facility and the destination

Care of the Nurses Who Are Grieving

- Caring long-term for a client can create personal attachments for nurses.

- Nurses can use coping strategies, such as:

  o Attending the client's funeral

  o Communicating in writing to the client's family

  o Attending debriefing sessions with colleagues

  o Using stress-management techniques

  o Talking with a professional counselor

CHAPTER 25: CARE OF THOSE WHO ARE DYING AND/OR GRIEVING

(A) Application Exercises

Scenario: A 68-year-old client, accompanied by her grown daughter, comes to the community mental health facility. She tells the nurse that her husband of 45 years died suddenly in a motor vehicle crash over 1 year ago. He ran into another car while under the influence of alcohol, killing both himself and a child passenger in the other car. Since that time, the client has been unable to continue any of her normal activities. She states that she has been too tired to even keep the house clean and has experienced long bouts of crying every day. She relates that she feels angry at her husband for drinking and for leaving her alone, since he was "supposed to be the one to take care of me!" The client relates that she only came to the mental health facility because her daughter was visiting from across the country and "made me come." The daughter says that the client seldom leaves the house and will not see her old friends.

1. Identify factors that put the client at risk for dysfunctional grieving.

2. What signs are present to indicate that this client's grief is becoming prolonged?

3. What further assessments should the nurse make at this time?

4. A nurse is caring for an older adult female client who was recently placed in a residential care facility by her three adult children. The client's spouse died 1 year ago, and the client is no longer able to care for herself. What assessment data should the nurse collect from the client's children?

5. A nurse is caring for a client who is dying. Identify three nursing interventions that the nurse can use to assist the client to maintain dignity and self-esteem during end-of-life care.

CHAPTER 25: CARE OF THOSE WHO ARE DYING AND/OR GRIEVING

(A) Application Exercises Answer Key

Scenario: A 68-year-old client, accompanied by her grown daughter, comes to the community mental health facility. She tells the nurse that her husband of 45 years died suddenly in a motor vehicle crash over 1 year ago. He ran into another car while under the influence of alcohol, killing both himself and a child passenger in the other car. Since that time, the client has been unable to continue any of her normal activities. She states that she has been too tired to even keep the house clean and has experienced long bouts of crying every day. She relates that she feels angry at her husband for drinking and for leaving her alone, since he was "supposed to be the one to take care of me!" The client relates that she only came to the mental health facility because her daughter was visiting from across the country and "made me come." The daughter says that the client seldom leaves the house and will not see her old friends.

1. Identify factors that put the client at risk for dysfunctional grieving.

> **Her husband died suddenly and violently in a motor vehicle crash while under the influence of alcohol.**

> **Her husband was also responsible for taking the life of a child as a result of the motor vehicle crash.**

> **There is a lack of social support, as the client has stopped seeing her friends, and her daughter lives far away.**

> **The client has stopped her usual activities and is socially isolated.**

 NCLEX® Connection: Psychosocial Integrity: Grief and Loss

2. What signs are present to indicate that this client's grief is becoming prolonged?

> **The client has bouts of crying every day and remains angry at her husband.**

> **The client exhibits behavior changes including fatigue and isolation.**

> **The client no longer sees her old friends.**

 NCLEX® Connection: Psychosocial Integrity: Grief and Loss

3. What further assessments should the nurse at this time?

> **Assess the client for suicidal ideation, depression, and anxiety.**

 NCLEX® Connection: Psychosocial Integrity: Grief and Loss

4. A nurse is caring for an older adult female client who was recently placed in a residential care facility by her three adult children. The client's spouse died 1 year ago, and the client is no longer able to care for herself. What assessment data should the nurse collect from the client's children?

> Previous coping strategies for each member of the family
>
> Family's cultural rituals, if any
>
> Family's religious/spiritual affiliations, if any
>
> Stage of grief in which each family member is involved with regard to the father's death and the mother's illness
>
> Current state of the mother's illness, and the family's understanding of it

 NCLEX® Connection: Psychosocial Integrity: Grief and Loss

5. A nurse is caring for a client who is dying. Identify three nursing interventions that the nurse can use to assist the client to maintain dignity and self-esteem during end-of-life care.

> Listen to the client's concerns.
>
> Maintain cleanliness and odor control in the client's physical environment.
>
> Allow the client to participate in ADLs as desired.
>
> Provide personal grooming assistance as necessary.
>
> Encourage the client to make decisions regarding food selection, activities, and health care.

 NCLEX® Connection: Psychosocial Integrity: End-of-Life Care

UNIT 5   SPECIAL POPULATIONS

Chapter 26   Mental Health Issues of Children and Adolescents

Overview

- Mental health and developmental disorders in children and adolescents are not always easily diagnosed, and treatment interventions may be delayed or inadequate. Factors that contribute to this include:

    ○ Children do not have the ability or the necessary skills to describe what is happening.

    ○ Children demonstrate a wide variation of "normal" behaviors, especially in different developmental stages.

    ○ It is difficult to determine if a child's behavior indicates an emotional problem.

- A child's behavior is problematic when it interferes with home, school, and interactions with peers.

    ○ Behaviors are considered pathologic when they

        ▪ Are not age appropriate.

        ▪ Deviate from cultural norms.

        ▪ Create deficits or impairments in adaptive functioning.

- Disorders that may appear during childhood and adolescence include:

    ○ Mood disorders, such as major depressive disorder, dysthymic disorder, bipolar disorder, including suicide

    ○ Anxiety disorders

    ○ Substance abuse, such as the abuse of cigarettes, alcohol, illegal drugs

    ○ Eating disorders, particularly among girls

    ○ Behavioral disorders, such as attention deficit hyperactivity disorder (ADHD), oppositional defiant disorder, and conduct disorder

    ○ Developmental disorders, such as an autistic disorder

- Childhood disorders may have associated comorbid conditions.

- The characteristics of good mental health for a child and adolescent include:

  - Ability to appropriately interpret reality, as well as having a correct perception of the surrounding environment

  - Positive self-concept

  - Ability to cope with stress and anxiety in an age-appropriate way

  - Mastery of developmental tasks

  - Ability to express oneself spontaneously and creatively

  - Ability to develop satisfying relationships

Assessment

- General Risk Factors

  - Genetic – Some disorders, such as schizophrenia, bipolar disorder, autism, ADHD, and certain causes of mental retardation may be associated with chromosomal abnormalities.

  - Biochemical – Alterations in neurotransmitters, including norepinephrine, serotonin, or dopamine, contribute to some mental disorders.

  - Social and environmental – Severe marital discord, low socioeconomic status, large families and overcrowding, parental criminality, substance abuse, maternal psychiatric disorders, foster care placement, physical and sexual abuse, and traumatic life events are all risk factors.

  - Cultural and ethnic – Difficulty with assimilation, lack of cultural role models, and lack of support from the dominant culture can contribute to mental health issues.

  - Resiliency – The ability to adapt to changes in the environment, form nurturing relationships, distance oneself from the emotional chaos of the parent or family, and use problem-solving skills can help an at-risk child develop normally.

  - Occurrence of traumatic events in the formative years is a risk factor.

Mood Disorders

- Risk factors associated with childhood depression include:

  - Family history of depression

  - Physical or sexual abuse or neglect

  - Homelessness

  - Disputes among parents, conflicts with peers or family, and rejection by peers or family

  - Engaging in high-risk behavior

- o Learning disabilities

- o Having a chronic illness

- Subjective and Objective Data

  - o Feelings of sadness

  - o Loss of appetite

  - o Nonspecific complaints related to health

  - o Engaging in solitary play or work

  - o Changes in appetite resulting in weight changes

  - o Changes in sleeping patterns

  - o Irritability

  - o Aggression

  - o High-risk behavior

  - o Poor school performance and/or dropping out of school

  - o Feelings of hopelessness about the future

  - o Suicidal tendencies.

Anxiety Disorders

- Subjective and Objective Data

  - o An anxiety disorder exists when the following occur:

    - ▪ The anxiety interferes with normal growth and development.

    - ▪ The anxiety is so serious that the child is unable to function normally at home, in school, and in other areas of life.

- Separation Anxiety Disorder

  - o This type of disorder is characterized by excessive anxiety when a child is separated from or anticipating separation from home or parents. The anxiety may develop into a school phobia or phobia of being left alone. Depression is also common.

  - o Anxiety may develop after a specific stressor (death of a relative or pet, an illness, a move, an assault).

  - o Anxiety may progress to a panic disorder or specific phobias.

- Posttraumatic Stress Disorder (PTSD)

  - o PTSD may be precipitated by experiencing or seeing a traumatic event.

  - o Children with PTSD may have psychologic symptoms of anxiety, depression, phobia, or conversion reactions.

- Children with PTSD will respond to the precipitating event in a series of phases. The phases begin with an arousal that lasts a few minutes to hours followed by a period of about 2 weeks in which the child will attempt to deal with the event using defense mechanisms. The last phase, lasting for a period of several months, is when the child may have psychologic symptoms as attempts are made to cope with the event. Failure to cope can lead to obsession regarding the event.

- If the anxiety resulting from PTSD is displayed externally, it may be manifested as irritability and aggression with family and friends, poor academic performance, somatic reports, belief that life will be short, and difficulty sleeping.

Behavior Disorders

- Subjective and Objective Data

  - Behavioral problems usually occur in school, church, home, and/or recreational activities.

  - In children with behavior disorders, symptoms generally worsen in the following:

    - Situations that require sustained attention

    - Unstructured group situations, such as the playground or classroom

- Attention deficit hyperactivity disorder (ADHD) involves the inability of a person to control behaviors requiring sustained attention.

  - Inattention, impulsivity, and hyperactivity are characteristic behaviors of ADHD.

    - Inattention is evidenced by a difficulty in paying attention, listening, and focusing.

    - Hyperactivity is evidenced by fidgeting, an inability to sit still, running and climbing inappropriately, difficulty with playing quietly, and talking excessively.

    - Impulsivity is evidenced by difficulty waiting for turns, constantly interrupting others, and acting without the consideration of consequences.

  - Inattentive or impulsive behavior may put the child at risk for injury.

  - Behaviors associated with ADHD must be present prior to age 7 and must be present in more than one setting to be diagnosed as ADHD. Behaviors associated with ADHD may receive negative attention from adults and peers.

  - Types of ADHD include:

    - Combined type – Most common

    - ADHD predominantly inattentive

    - ADHD predominantly hyperactive-impulsive

- Oppositional Defiant Disorder

  - This disorder is characterized by a recurrent pattern of the following antisocial behaviors:

    - Negativity

    - Disobedience

    - Hostility

    - Defiant behaviors (especially toward authority figures)

    - Stubbornness

    - Argumentativeness

    - Limit testing

    - Unwillingness to compromise

    - Refusal to accept responsibility for misbehavior

  - Misbehavior is usually demonstrated at home and directed toward the person best known.

  - Children and adolescents who have oppositional defiant disorder do not see themselves as defiant. They view their behavior as a response to unreasonable demands and/or circumstances.

  - Clients with this behavior disorder may exhibit low self-esteem, mood lability, and a low frustration threshold.

  - Oppositional defiant disorder can develop into conduct disorder.

- Conduct Disorder

CONTRIBUTING FACTORS	MANIFESTATIONS
• Parental rejection and neglect • Difficult infant temperament • Inconsistent child-rearing practices with harsh discipline • Physical or sexual abuse • Lack of supervision • Early institutionalization • Frequent changing of caregivers • Large family size • Association with delinquent peer groups • Parent with a history of psychological illness	• Demonstrates a lack of remorse or care for the feelings of others • Bullies, threatens, and intimidates others • Believes that aggression is justified • Exhibits low self-esteem, irritability, temper outbursts, reckless behavior • May demonstrate signs of suicidal ideation • May have concurrent learning disorders or impairments in cognitive functioning • Demonstrates physical cruelty to others and/or animals • Has used a weapon that could cause serious injuries • Destroys property of others • Has run away from home • Often lies, shoplifts, and is truant from school

- Pervasive Developmental Disorders

  o Autism

    - Autism is complex neurodevelopmental disorder believed to be of genetic origin with a wide spectrum of behaviors affecting an individual's ability to communicate and interact with others. Cognitive and language development are typically delayed. Characteristic behaviors include inability to maintain eye contact, repetitive actions, and strict observance of routines.

    - This type of disorder is usually observed before 3 years of age.

    - Physical difficulties experienced by the child with autism include sensory integration dysfunction, sleep disorders, digestive disorders, feeding disorders, epilepsy, and/or allergies.

    - There is a wide variability in functioning. Abilities may range from poor (inability to perform self-care, inability to communicate and relate to others) to high (ability to function at near normal levels).

- Other disorders seen in children include:

  o Mental retardation

    - Below-average intellectual functioning as measured by an IQ less than 70

    - Significant limitations in communication, self-care, home living, self-direction, social skills, community use, work, leisure, academic achievement, health, and safety

  o Learning disorders

    - Group of disorders characterized by difficulty in gaining and using essential skills of listening and speaking

    - Treated through special education

  o Communication disorders

    - May be expressive, receptive, or a combination of both

    - Treated through a variety of modalities, examples of which include speech and language therapies, adaptive communication devices, hearing aids, and sign language

Collaborative Care

- Nursing Care

  o Obtain a complete nursing history to include the following:

    - Mother's pregnancy and birth history.

    - Sleeping, eating, and elimination patterns; recent weight loss or gain.

    - Achievement of developmental milestones.

    - Allergies.

- Current medications.
- Peer and family relationships, school performance.
- History of emotional, physical, or sexual abuse.
- Parent's perceptions and level of tolerance toward child's behavior.
- Family history, including current members of the household.
- Substance use/abuse.
    - □ Tobacco products, such as cigarettes, cigars, snuff, chewing tobacco
    - □ Alcohol, frequency of use, driving under the influence, and family history of abuse
    - □ Drugs (illegal or prescription) to get high, stay calm, lose weight, or stay awake
- Safety at home and at school
- Actual or potential risk for self-injury
- Presence of depression and suicidal ideation, including a plan, the lethality of that plan, and the means to carry out the plan
- Availability of weapons in the home

- ○ Perform a complete physical assessment, including a mental status examination.
- ○ Use primary prevention, such as education, peer group discussions, and mentoring to prevent risky behavior and to promote healthy behavior and effective coping.
    - Work with clients to adopt a realistic view of their bodies and to improve overall self-esteem.
    - Identify and reinforce the use of positive coping skills.
    - Employ the use of gun and weapon control strategies.
    - Emphasize the use of seat belts when in motor vehicles.
    - Encourage the use of protective gear for high-impact sports.
    - Provide education on contraceptives and other sexual information, such as the transmission and prevention of HIV and other sexually transmitted diseases.
    - Encourage abstinence, but keep the lines of communication open to allow the adolescent to discuss sexual practices.
    - Encourage clients and family members to seek professional help if indicated.
- ○ Intervene for clients who have engaged in high-risk behaviors.
    - Instruct the client and family on factors that contribute to substance dependency and tobacco use. Make appropriate referrals when indicated.
    - Inform the client and family about support groups in the community for eating disorders, substance abuse, and general teen support.

- Instruct the client regarding individuals within the school environment and community to whom concerns can be voiced about personal safety, such as police officers, school nurses, counselors, teachers.

- Make referrals to social services when indicated.

- Discuss the use and availability of support hotlines.

- Perform a depression and suicide assessment. Make an immediate referral for professional care when indicated.

  o Cognitive-behavioral therapy is useful to change negative thoughts to positive outcomes when intervening for depression.

  o Interventions for anxiety disorders include:

  - Providing emotional support that is accepting of regression and other defense mechanisms

  - Offering protection during panic levels of anxiety by providing for needs

  - Implementing methods to increase client self-esteem and feelings of achievement

  - Providing assistance with working through traumatic events or losses to reach an acceptance of what has happened

  - Encouraging group therapy

- Interventions for Behavior Disorders:

  o Use a calm, firm, respectful approach with the child.

  o Use modeling to show acceptable behavior.

  o Obtain the child's attention before giving directions. Provide short and clear explanations.

  o Set clear limits on unacceptable behaviors and be consistent.

  o Plan physical activities through which the child can use energy and obtain success.

  o Assist parents to develop a reward system using methods, such as a wall chart or tokens. Encourage the child to participate.

  o Focus on the family and child's strengths, not just the problems.

  o Support the parents' efforts to remain hopeful.

  o Provide a safe environment for the child and others.

  o Provide the child with specific positive feedback when expectations are met.

  o Identify issues that result in power struggles.

  o Assist the child in developing effective coping mechanisms.

  o Encourage the child to participate in group, individual, and family therapy.

  o Administer medications, such as antipsychotics, mood stabilizers, anticonvulsants, and antidepressants; monitor for side effects.

- Interventions for an Autism Spectrum Disorder:

  - Initiate a referral for early intervention

  - Provide for a structured environment.

  - Consult with parents to provide consistent and individualized care.

  - Encourage parents to participate and remain at the bedside as much as possible.

  - Use short, concise, and developmentally appropriate communication.

  - Identify desired behaviors and reward them.

  - Role model social skills.

  - Role play situations that involve conflict.

  - Encourage verbal communication.

  - Limit self-stimulating and ritualistic behaviors by providing alternative play activities.

  - Determine emotional and situational triggers.

  - Give plenty of notice before changing routines.

  - Carefully monitor the child's behaviors to ensure safety.

- Medications

  - Medications for children and adolescents include selective serotonin reuptake inhibitors, such as fluoxetine (Prozac); tricyclic antidepressants such as amitriptyline (Elavil); atypical anxiolytic, such as buspirone (BuSpar); CNS stimulants, such as methylphenidate (Concerta, Ritalin SR); and norepinephrine selective reuptake inhibitors, such as atomoxetine HCl (Strattera).

- Client Outcomes

  - The client achieves maximal level of physical, cognitive, and social development.

  - The client is able to communicate effectively.

  - The child and family verbalize the need for information and support.

  - The client verbalizes improved mood.

  - The client develops realistic goals for the future.

  - The family identifies strategies for managing disruptive or inappropriate behaviors.

  - The family identifies strategies for managing long-term care of the child.

CHAPTER 26: MENTAL HEALTH ISSUES OF CHILDREN AND ADOLESCENTS

Ⓐ Application Exercises

Scenario: A 15 year old comes into the school health clinic reporting a stomachache. The nurse notices that she makes little eye contact when answering questions and has superficial scratches on her right wrist. The student appears underweight and emotionally distant. She states that her parents have recently divorced and that she just moved to this school district. She says, "I miss my boyfriend and friends from my old school."

1. What key areas should the nurse assess with this student?

2. When assessing this adolescent for depression, which of the following findings should the nurse expect? (Select all that apply.)

    _____   Insomnia

    _____   Feelings of sadness

    _____   Increased activity level

    _____   Irritability

    _____   Aggressiveness

3. The student tells the nurse that, "Nothing is fun anymore; it just doesn't seem worth the effort." How should the nurse respond?

4. A 5 year old is brought to a mental health agency by his mother. The mother says the child is unable to sit through meals and is so easily distracted that he cannot even sit through a 30-min cartoon video. His kindergarten teacher reports difficulty following directions and attending to one task. The nurse should recognize that these findings are consistent with

    A. mental retardation.

    B. oppositional defiant disorder.

    C. posttraumatic stress disorder.

    D. attention deficit hyperactivity disorder.

5. A 12-year-old child demonstrates signs and symptoms of conduct disorder. These include which of the following manifestations? (Select all that apply.)

    _____   Hostility

    _____   Frequent lying

    _____   Breaking of objects due to impulsiveness

    _____   Law-breaking activities

    _____   Careless mistakes

    _____   Cruelty to neighborhood pets

    _____   Poor eye contact with others

6. A nurse is assessing a 4-year-old child for signs of autism. The nurse should be alert for

    A. constant talking and impulsive behavior.

    B. poor language and interpersonal skills.

    C. destructiveness and history of irritability and hostility.

    D. night terrors and reports of somatic problems.

CHAPTER 26: MENTAL HEALTH ISSUES OF CHILDREN AND ADOLESCENTS

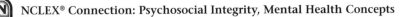

(A) Application Exercises Answer Key

Scenario: A 15 year old comes into the school health clinic reporting a stomachache. The nurse notices that she makes little eye contact when answering questions and has superficial scratches on her right wrist. The student appears underweight and emotionally distant. She states that her parents have recently divorced and that she just moved to this school district. She says, "I miss my boyfriend and friends from my old school."

1. What key areas should the nurse assess with this student?

> **Dietary intake**
>
> **History of weight loss**
>
> **Peer relationships at new school**
>
> **Current contact with boyfriend or friends at previous school**
>
> **Feelings of safety at home and school**
>
> **Actual or potential self-injury**
>
> **Feelings of depression**
>
> **History of sexual activity, including possibility of pregnancy**
>
> **Substance use (alcohol, drugs, tobacco products)**
>
> **History of abuse (physical, emotional, sexual)**
>
> **Current history of academic performance and school involvement**

(N) NCLEX® Connection: Psychosocial Integrity, Mental Health Concepts

2. When assessing this adolescent for depression, which of the following findings should the nurse expect? (Select all that apply.)

> _____ Insomnia
>
> __X__   **Feelings of sadness**
>
> _____ Increased activity level
>
> __X__   **Irritability**
>
> __X__   **Aggressiveness**

Signs and symptoms of depression may include feelings of sadness, irritability and aggressiveness. An adolescent with depression is more likely to experience hypersomnia and psychomotor retardation.

(N) NCLEX® Connection: Psychosocial Integrity, Mental Health Concepts

3. The student tells the nurse that, "Nothing is fun anymore; it just doesn't seem worth the effort." How should the nurse respond?

> The nurse should ask the student to clarify what she means by, "It just doesn't seem worth the effort." Specifically, the nurse should ask if she has thoughts of hurting herself. If the teen states that she is thinking of suicide, the nurse needs to determine if she has a plan, what the plan is, the lethality of the plan, and the availability of the means to carry out the plan (e.g., guns in the home). The nurse should make an immediate referral for professional care based on the student's response. The nurse should stay with the student at all times until placement and offer support through listening and acceptance.

 NCLEX® Connection: Psychosocial Integrity, Therapeutic Communications

4. A 5 year old is brought to a mental health agency by his mother. The mother says the child is unable to sit through meals and is so easily distracted that he cannot even sit through a 30-min cartoon video. His kindergarten teacher reports difficulty following directions and attending to one task. The nurse should recognize that these findings are consistent with

   A. mental retardation.

   B. oppositional defiant disorder.

   C. posttraumatic stress disorder.

   D. attention deficit hyperactivity disorder.

> ADHD is characterized by constant movement, distractibility, and difficulty focusing on tasks. Mental retardation is evidenced by below average intellectual functioning as measured by an IQ less than 70. If oppositional defiant disorder were the problem, the child would be argumentative and push the limits of parental authority. PTSD is characterized by aggressiveness, somatic reports, and irritability.

 NCLEX® Connection: Psychosocial Integrity, Mental Health Concepts

5. A 12-year-old child demonstrates signs and symptoms of conduct disorder. These include which of the following manifestations? (Select all that apply.)

   __X__   **Hostility**

   __X__   **Frequent lying**

   _____   Breaking of objects due to impulsiveness

   __X__   **Law-breaking activities**

   _____   Careless mistakes

   __X__   **Cruelty to neighborhood pets**

   _____   Poor eye contact with others

> Hostility, telling lies, breaking laws, and cruelty to animals are all manifestations common in conduct disorder. Breaking objects and making careless mistakes are more likely related to ADHD. Poor eye contact is more likely a manifestation of autism.

 NCLEX® Connection: Psychosocial Integrity, Mental Health Concepts

6. A nurse is assessing a 4-year-old child for signs of autism. The nurse should be alert for

    A. constant talking and impulsive behavior.

    B. poor language and interpersonal skills.

    C. destructiveness and history of irritability and hostility.

    D. night terrors and reports of somatic problems.

Children with autism have difficulty learning language skills and may fail to develop interpersonal relationships. Constant talking and impulsive behavior are among the signs of ADHD. Destructiveness, irritability, and hostility relate to conduct disorder. Night terrors and somatic problems relate to PTSD.

Ⓝ NCLEX® Connection: Psychosocial Integrity, Mental Health Concepts

UNIT 6: PSYCHIATRIC EMERGENCIES

- Crisis Management
- Suicide
- Anger Management
- Family and Community Violence
- Sexual Assault

NCLEX® CONNECTIONS

When reviewing the chapters in this unit, keep in mind the relevant sections of the NCLEX® outline, in particular:

CLIENT NEEDS: PSYCHOSOCIAL INTEGRITY

Relevant topics/tasks include:
- Crisis Intervention
  - Identify a client in crisis.
  - Use crisis intervention techniques to assist the client in coping.
  - Apply knowledge of client psychopathology to crisis intervention.

UNIT 6	PSYCHIATRIC EMERGENCIES
Chapter 27	Crisis Management

Overview

- A crisis is an acute, time-limited (usually lasting 4 to 6 weeks) event during which a client experiences an emotional response that cannot be managed with the client's normal coping mechanisms.

- Common characteristics include:

    o Experience of a sudden event with little or no time to prepare

    o Perception of the event as life threatening

    o Loss or decrease in communication with significant others

    o Sense of displacement from the familiar

    o An actual or perceived loss

- Types of crises include:

    o Situational/external – often unanticipated loss or change experienced in every day, often unanticipated, life events

    o Maturational/internal – achieving new developmental stages, which requires learning additional coping mechanisms

    o Adventitious – the occurrence of natural disasters, crimes, or national disasters

Assessment

- Risk and Protective Factors

    o Accumulation of unresolved losses

    o Current life stressors

    o Concurrent mental and physical health issues

    o Excessive fatigue or pain

    o Age and developmental stage

    o Support system

    o Prior experience with stress/crisis

- Subjective/Objective Data
  - The nursing history should include the following:
    - Presence of suicidal or homicidal ideation requiring hospitalization
    - The client's perception of the precipitating event
    - Cultural or religious needs of the client
    - Support system
    - Present coping skills
  - Phases of a crisis

PHASE	MANIFESTATIONS
Phase 1	Escalating anxiety from a threat activates increased defense responses.
Phase 2	Anxiety continues escalating as defense responses fail, functioning becomes disorganized, and the client resorts to trial-and-error attempts to resolve anxiety.
Phase 3	Trial-and-error methods of resolution fail, and the client's anxiety escalates to severe or panic levels, leading to flight or withdrawal behaviors.
Phase 4	The client experiences overwhelming anxiety that can lead to anguish and apprehension, feelings of powerlessness and being overwhelmed, dissociative symptoms (depersonalization, detachment from reality), depression, confusion, and/or violence against others or self.

Collaborative Care

- Nursing Care
  - Initial interventions include:
    - Identifying the current problem and directing interventions for resolution
    - Taking an active, directive role with the client
    - Helping the client to set realistic, attainable goals
  - Provide for client safety.
    - Initiate hospitalization to protect clients with suicidal or homicidal thoughts.
    - Prioritize interventions to address the client's physical needs first.
  - Use strategies to decrease anxiety.
    - Develop a therapeutic nurse-client relationship.
      - Remain with the client
      - Listen and observe.
      - Make eye contact.
      - Ask questions related to the client's feelings.

- ▫ Ask questions related to the event.

- ▫ Demonstrate genuineness and caring.

- ▫ Communicate clearly and, if needed, with clear directives.

- ▫ Avoid false reassurance and other nontherapeutic responses.

- ○ Teach relaxation techniques, such as meditation.

- ○ Identify and teach coping skills (assertiveness training, parenting skills, occupational training).

- ○ Assist the client with the development of the following type of action plan:

  - ▪ Short-term, no longer than 24 to 72 hr

  - ▪ Focused on the crisis

  - ▪ Realistic and manageable

- Medications

  - ○ Administer antianxiety and/or antidepressant medication as prescribed.

- Client Education

  - ○ Identify and coordinate with support agencies and other resources.

  - ○ Plan and provide for follow-up care.

- Client Outcomes

  - ○ Client is able to make decisions between two or more options.

  - ○ Client is able to manage anxiety with relaxation techniques.

  - ○ Client returns to precrisis level of functioning.

CHAPTER 27: CRISIS MANAGEMENT

 Application Exercises

Scenario: A client is being seen in the emergency department after a motor vehicle crash in which a drunk driver crashed into the passenger's side of the client's car. The client was trapped in the wreckage next to his adolescent son, who did not survive the impact. The client has lacerations requiring sutures, moderate blood loss, and a broken arm, but he was not seriously injured. The nurse notices that, despite being informed that his son has died, the client continues to ask about the son's well-being, and seems confused when attempting to answer simple questions.

1. What is the priority nursing intervention for this client?

2. Which phase of crisis is this client experiencing? What assessment data confirm this?

3. Identify initial nursing interventions appropriate for this client.

4. What type of crisis did this client experience?

5. Which of the following medications might be prescribed for a client experiencing a crisis? (Select all that apply.)

    _____   Lithium carbonate (Lithobid)

    _____   Paroxetine (Paxil)

    _____   Risperidone (Risperdal)

    _____   Haloperidol (Haldol)

    _____   Lorazepam (Ativan)

CHAPTER 27: CRISIS MANAGEMENT

 Application Exercises Answer Key

Scenario: A client is being seen in the emergency department after a motor vehicle crash in which a drunk driver crashed into the passenger's side of the client's car. The client was trapped in the wreckage next to his adolescent son, who did not survive the impact. The client has lacerations requiring sutures, moderate blood loss, and a broken arm, but he was not seriously injured. The nurse notices that, despite being informed that his son has died, the client continues to ask about the son's well-being, and seems confused when attempting to answer simple questions.

1. What is the priority nursing intervention for this client?

The priority nursing intervention for this client is safety. He should be assessed for suicidal or homicidal ideation.

 NCLEX® Connection: Psychosocial Integrity: Crisis Intervention

2. Which phase of crisis is this client experiencing? What assessment data confirm this?

Phase 4: The client is experiencing overwhelming anxiety that can lead to anguish, apprehension, depression, confusion and/or violence against others or himself. The client is unable to answer simple questions and does not seem to understand the reality of his son's death. He may be experiencing dissociative symptoms, such as depersonalization or detachment from reality.

 NCLEX® Connection: Psychosocial Integrity: Crisis Intervention

3. Identify initial nursing interventions appropriate for this client.

Stay with the client; listen, observe, and ask questions based on cues from him.

Notify the appropriate support system in the facility, such as a chaplain, social workers, and/ or trained volunteers.

Question the client about family support and ask other members of the health care team to notify them.

Prioritize care starting with the client's immediate physical needs.

 NCLEX® Connection: Psychosocial Integrity: Crisis Intervention

4. What type of crisis did this client experience?

Situational: unanticipated loss in an external life event

 NCLEX® Connection: Psychosocial Integrity: Crisis Intervention

5. Which of the following medications might be prescribed for a client experiencing a crisis? (Select all that apply.)

_____ Lithium carbonate (Lithobid)

__X__ **Paroxetine (Paxil)**

_____ Risperidone (Risperdal)

_____ Haloperidol (Haldol)

__X__ **Lorazepam (Ativan)**

Antidepressants are most likely to be prescribed for the depression that may follow a crisis situation. Mood stabilizers are used for bipolar disorder. Antipsychotic medications may be prescribed for disturbed thought processes, usually when accompanied by other psychotic symptoms (hallucinations, delusions, blunt affect). Antipsychotics are not indicated in a short-term crisis situation. A benodiazepine may be useful to minimize the anxiety that a client might fell in a crisis situation.

NCLEX® Connection: Pharmacological and Parenteral Therapies: Expected Effects/Outcomes

UNIT 6	PSYCHIATRIC EMERGENCIES
Chapter 28	Suicide

Overview

- Suicide is the intentional act of killing oneself.

- A client who is suicidal may be ambivalent about death; intervention can make a difference.

- A client contemplating suicide believes that the act is the end to problems. Little concern is given to the aftermath and the ramifications to those left behind. Long-term therapy is needed for the survivors.

- Suicidal ideation occurs when a client is having thoughts about committing suicide.

- Myths regarding suicide include:

  o People who talk about suicide never commit it.

  o People who are suicidal only want to hurt themselves, not others.

  o There is no way to help someone who really wants to kill himself.

  o Mention of the word suicide will cause the suicidal individual to actually commit suicide.

  o Ignoring verbal threats of suicide, or challenging a person to carry out suicide plans, will reduce the individual's use of these behaviors.

  o People who talk about suicide are only trying to get attention.

- Levels of Nursing Intervention

  o Primary – prevention strategies that include providing information and education to at-risk populations

  o Secondary – management of the suicide crisis

Assessment

- Risk Factors

  o Those at highest risk for suicide include adolescent, young adult, and older adult males; Native Americans as a group; and persons with comorbid mental illness, such as depressive disorders, anxiety disorders, substance abuse, schizophrenia, and personality disorders.

Ⓖ

     ○   Untreated depression increases the risk of suicide in the older adult client. Other risk factors for the older adult client include: loss of employment and finances, feelings of isolation, powerlessness, prior attempts at suicide (Older adult clients are more likely to succeed.), change in functional ability, alcohol or other substance abuse, loss of loved ones.

     ○   Biological factors include:

           ■   Family history of suicide

           ■   Physical disorders, such as AIDS, cancer, cardiovascular disease, stroke, chronic renal failure, cirrhosis, dementia, epilepsy, head injury, Huntington's disease, and multiple sclerosis

     ○   Psychosocial factors include:

           ■   Sense of hopelessness

           ■   Intense emotions, such as rage, anger, or guilt

           ■   Poor interpersonal relationships at home and work

           ■   Developmental stressors, such as those experienced by adolescents

- Protective Factors

     ○   Feelings of responsibility toward family

     ○   Current pregnancy

     ○   Religious and cultural beliefs

     ○   Overall satisfaction with life

     ○   Presence of adequate social support

     ○   Effective coping and problem-solving skills

     ○   Access to appropriate medical care

- Subjective Data

     ○   Assess carefully for verbal and nonverbal clues. It is important to ask the client if he is thinking of suicide. This will not give the client the idea to commit suicide.

     ○   Comments are usually made to someone that the client perceives as supportive.

     ○   Comments or signals may be overt or covert.

           ■   Overt comment – "There is just no reason for me to go on living."

           ■   Covert comment – "Everything is looking pretty grim for me."

- o   Assess the client's suicide plan:
    - ▪   How lethal is the plan?
    - ▪   Can the client describe the plan exactly?
    - ▪   Does the client have access to the intended method?
    - ▪   Has the client's mood changed? A sudden change in mood from sad and depressed to happy and peaceful may indicate a client's intention to commit suicide.
- •   Objective Data
    - o   Lacerations, scratches, and scars that could indicate previous attempts at self-harm
- •   Standardized Assessment Tool
    - o   The SAD PERSONS scale is a valuable tool that assesses 10 major risk factors for suicide and assigns scores for each.

Collaborative Care

- •   Nursing Care
    - o   Self-assessment
        - ▪   The nurse must determine how she feels personally about suicide.
        - ▪   The nurse must become comfortable asking personal questions about suicidal ideation and following up on client's answers.
        - ▪   Death of a client by suicide can cause health care professionals to experience a hopelessness, helplessness, ambivalence, anger, anxiety, avoidance, and denial.
    - o   Suicide precautions include milieu therapy within the facility.
        - ▪   Initiate one-on-one constant supervision around the clock, always having the client in sight and close.
        - ▪   Document the client's location, mood, quoted statements, and behavior every 15 min or per facility protocol.
        - ▪   Remove all glass, metal silverware, electrical cords, vases, belts, shoelaces, metal nail files, tweezers, matches, razors, perfume, shampoo, and plastic bags from the client's room and vicinity.
        - ▪   Allow the client to use only plastic eating utensils.
        - ▪   Check the environment for possible hazards (such as windows that open, overhead pipes that are easily accessible.)
        - ▪   During observation periods, always check the client's hands, especially if they are hidden from sight.

- Ensure that the client swallows all medications.

- Identify whether or not the client's current medications can be lethal with overdose. If so, collaborate with the provider to have less dangerous medications substituted if possible.

- Ensure that visitors are aware of suicide precautions and rules restricting bringing possibly harmful items to the client.

○ Therapeutic communication

- When questioning the client about suicide, always use a follow-up question if the first answer is negative. For example: the client says, "I'm feeling completely hopeless." The nurse says, "Are you thinking of suicide?" Client: "No, I'm just sad." Nurse: "I can see you're very sad. Are you thinking about hurting yourself?" Client: "Well, I've thought about it a lot."

- Establish a trusting therapeutic relationship.

- Limit the amount of time an at-risk client spends alone.

- Involve significant others in the treatment plan.

- Carry out treatment plans for the client with comorbid disorders, such as a dual diagnosis of substance abuse.

○ Medications to prevent suicide include:

CLASSIFICATION	MEDICATION EXAMPLE	CLIENT TEACHING
Antidepressants: Selective Serotonin Reuptake Inhibitors (SSRIs)	• Citalopram (Celexa) • Fluoxetine (Prozac) • Sertraline (Zoloft)	• Do not stop taking medication suddenly. • Medications may take 1 to 3 weeks for therapeutic effects for initial response with up to 2 months for maximal response. • Avoid hazardous activities (driving, operating heavy equipment/machinery) until medication side effects are known. Side effects may include nausea, headache, and CNS stimulation (agitation, insomnia, anxiety). • Sexual dysfunction may occur. Notify the provider if effects are intolerable. • Follow a healthy diet, as weight gain can occur with long-term use. • Monitor for signs of increased depression and intent of suicide.

CLASSIFICATION	MEDICATION EXAMPLE	CLIENT TEACHING
Sedative Hypnotic Anxiolytics (Benzodiazepines)	• Diazepam (Valium) • Lorazepam (Ativan)	• Observe for CNS depression, such as sedation, lightheadedness, ataxia, and decreased cognitive function. • Avoid the use of other CNS depressants, such as alcohol. • Avoid hazardous activities (driving, operating heavy equipment/machinery). • Caffeine interferes with the desired effects of the medication. • Advise the client who has been taking these medications regularly and in high doses to taper the dose over several weeks to prevent withdrawal symptoms.
Mood stabilizers	Lithium carbonate (Eskalith)	• Gastrointestinal effects may be minimized by taking medication with food or milk. • Maintain a healthy diet, and exercise regularly to minimize weight gain. • Maintain fluid intake of 2 to 3 L/day from food and beverage sources. • Maintain adequate sodium intake. • Encourage the client to comply with laboratory appointments needed to monitor lithium effectiveness and adverse effects.
Antiepileptics	Valproic acid (Depakote)	• Take medication with food to minimize gastrointestinal discomfort.
Atypical antipsychotics	• Risperidone (Risperdal) • Olanzapine (Zyprexa)	• To minimize weight gain, advise the client to maintain a healthy diet and exercise regularly. • Instruct the client to report symptoms of agitation, dizziness, sedation, and sleep disruption to the provider, as the medication may need to be changed.

- Care After Discharge

  - Nursing Actions

    - Create a support-system list – Specific names, agencies, and telephone numbers that the client can call for support (especially important if the client is not in an acute care setting).

    - Ask the client to agree to a no-suicide contract, which is a verbal or written agreement that the client makes to not harm himself, but instead to seek help.

      - A no-suicide contract is not legally binding and should only be used according to agency policy.

      - A no-suicide contract may be beneficial, but it should not replace other suicide prevention strategies.

      - A no-suicide contract can be used as a tool to develop and maintain trust between the nurse and the client.

      - A no-suicide contract are discouraged for clients who are in crisis, under the influence of substances, psychotic, very impulsive, and/or very angry/agitated. A contract does not take the place of suicide precautions.

- Client Education

  - Assist the client to develop a support-system list with specific names, agencies, and telephone numbers that the client can call in case of an emergency.

- Client Outcomes

  - Client identifies at least two people who can provide emotional support.

  - Client verbalizes a decrease in anxiety.

  - Client remains free from harm.

CHAPTER 28: SUICIDE

 Application Exercises

Scenario: A nurse is working with a young adult male client who is single. The client was committed involuntarily 1 week ago to an acute care mental health facility. He has been diagnosed with bipolar disorder and has a recent history of alcohol abuse. The client ran away from home as a teenager and has been living on city streets ever since. He states that he was raised Roman Catholic and is still very religious. At the time of admission, he had been found intoxicated and ranting about being kidnapped by space creatures. He has a history of one previous suicide attempt by hanging.

1. Describe the client's risk factors, as well as any protective factors.

2. The nurse and the client are standing near a window on the sixth floor of the mental health facility. During this time, the client is lucid with no sign of psychosis and remarks, "I wonder if anyone has ever jumped from up here." How should the nurse reply?

3. The client shows willingness to talk to the nurse about current feelings but states, "I'll talk to you, but please, please don't tell anyone else what I am going to tell you now! Will you promise me?" What should the nurse do first?

4. The client describes a suicide plan with intent to carry out the plan while in the mental health facility, rather than at home, so he will not be found by family or friends. The client is immediately placed on suicide precautions. What should suicide precautions involve for this client?

5. A nurse assesses a client at a community mental health facility using the SAD PERSONS tool. The nurse knows that this tool provides which of the following data related to a client?

    A. Current anxiety level

    B. Problem-solving ability

    C. Suicide potential

    D. Mood disturbance

6. A client says, "I plan to commit suicide." Which of the following should be the nurse's priority assessment?

    A. Client's educational and economic background

    B. Lethality of the method and availability of means

    C. Quality of the client's social support

    D. Client's insight into the reasons for the decision

CHAPTER 28: SUICIDE

 Application Exercises Answer Key

Scenario: A nurse is working with a young adult male client who is single. The client was committed involuntarily 1 week ago to an acute care mental health facility. He has been diagnosed with bipolar disorder and has a recent history of alcohol abuse. The client ran away from home as a teenager and has been living on city streets ever since. He states that he was raised Roman Catholic and is still very religious. At the time of admission, he had been found intoxicated and ranting about being kidnapped by space creatures. He has a history of one previous suicide attempt by hanging.

1. Describe the client's risk factors, as well as any protective factors.

>   **Risk factors:**
>
>>   Single, young adult male
>>   History of bipolar disorder and recent substance abuse
>>   Disturbed thought processes on admission
>>   Previous suicide attempts using a lethal method
>>   Lack of family support system
>
>   **Protective factors:**
>
>>   Religious background

 NCLEX® Connection: Psychosocial Integrity: Crisis Intervention

2. The nurse and the client are standing near a window on the sixth floor of the mental health facility. During this time, the client is lucid with no sign of psychosis and remarks, "I wonder if anyone has ever jumped from up here." How should the nurse reply?

>   **The nurse should assess the client's suicidal ideation with a question such as, "Why do you ask? Are you thinking about harming yourself in that way?" If the answer is negative, the nurse should rephrase the question and ask it again.**

 NCLEX® Connection: Psychosocial Integrity: Crisis Intervention

3. The client shows willingness to talk to the nurse about current feelings but states, "I'll talk to you, but please, please don't tell anyone else what I am going to tell you now! Will you promise me?" What should the nurse do first?

>   **The nurse should tell the client that she cannot keep a secret that is related to the client's safety and welfare. The nurse is required to talk to the health care team about something so important. The nurse should make it clear that he cares about what happens to the client, and invite the client to sit down and talk.**

 NCLEX® Connection: Psychosocial Integrity, Crisis Intervention

4. The client describes a suicide plan with intent to carry out the plan while in the mental health facility, rather than at home, so he will not be found by family or friends. The client is immediately placed on suicide precautions. What should suicide precautions involve for this client?

The client is not only exhibiting suicidal ideation, but he also has a plan for carrying out the suicide. The client should be on one-to-one supervision by a staff member at all times. The milieu of the acute care mental health facility should already be free of most potentially harmful objects, but the nurse should make sure that this client's immediate environment is checked for possible harmful objects (shoelaces, belt, plastic bags). Collaboration with the client's treatment team is vital to ensure that a specific plan is in place to keep the client safe.

 NCLEX® Connection: Psychosocial Integrity, Crisis Intervention

5. A nurse assesses a client at a community mental health facility using the SAD PERSONS tool. The nurse knows that this tool provides which of the following data related to a client?

    A. Current anxiety level

    B. Problem-solving ability

    C. Suicide potential

    D. Mood disturbance

The SAD PERSONS tool is used specifically to assess the client's potential for committing suicide. Information on the other options is not provided by this tool.

 NCLEX® Connection: Psychosocial Integrity, Crisis Intervention

6. A client says, "I plan to commit suicide." Which of the following should be the nurse's priority assessment?

    A. Client's educational and economic background

    B. Lethality of method and availability of means

    C. Quality of the client's social support

    D. Client's insight into the reasons for the decision

The greatest risk to the client is self-harm as a result of carrying out a suicide plan. Therefore, the priority assessment is to determine how lethal the method is, how available the method is, and how detailed the plan is. Assessing the client's education and economic background, the quality of the client's social support, and the client's insight into the reasons for the decision are all important to care for this client, but they are not the priority assessments at this time.

 NCLEX® Connection: Psychosocial Integrity, Crisis Intervention

UNIT 6   PSYCHIATRIC EMERGENCIES

Chapter 29   Anger Management

Overview

- Anger, a normal feeling, is an emotional response to frustration as perceived by the individual. It can be positive if there is truly an unfair or wrong situation that needs to be righted.

- Anger becomes negative when it is denied, suppressed, or expressed inappropriately, such as by using aggressive behavior.

  o Denied or suppressed anger can manifest as physical or psychological symptoms, such as headaches, coronary artery disease, hypertension, gastric ulcers, depression, or low self-esteem.

- Aggression

  o Inappropriately expressed anger can become hostility or aggression.

  o Aggression includes physical or verbal responses that indicate rage and potential harm to self, others, or property.

  o A client who is often angry and aggressive may have underlying feelings of inadequacy, insecurity, guilt, fear, and rejection.

- Comorbidities include depressive disorders, PTSD, Alzheimer's disease, and personality and psychotic disorders.

- Categories/Taxonomies of Disorder

  o Preassaultive – The client begins to become angry and exhibits increasing anxiety, hyperactivity, and verbal abuse.

  o Assaultive – The client commits an act of violence. Seclusion and physical restraints may be required.

  o Postassaultive – Staff reviews the incident with the client during this stage.

- Despite the potential for anger and aggression among individuals with mental illness, it is important to know that individuals who are mentally ill are more likely to hurt themselves than to express aggression against others.

- Seclusion and restraint must be used only according to legal guidelines and should be the interventions of last resort after other less restrictive options have been tried.

  o Seclusion and restraint do not usually lead to positive behavior change. Seclusion and restraint may keep individuals safe during a violent outburst, but the use of restraint itself can be dangerous and has, on rare occasions, led to the death of clients due to reasons such as suffocation and strangulation.

  o Intramuscular medication may need to be given if aggression is threatening and if no medications were previously given.

  o Remove the client from seclusion or restraint as soon as the crisis is over and when the client attempts reconciliation and is no longer aggressive.

Assessment

- Risk Factors

  o Past history of aggression, poor impulse control, and violence

  o Poor coping skills, limited support systems

  o Comorbidity that leads to acts of violence (psychotic delusions, command hallucinations, violent angry reactions with cognitive disorders)

  o Living in a violent environment

  o Limit setting by the nurse within the therapeutic milieu

- Subjective and Objective Data

  o Hyperactivity such as pacing, restlessness

  o Defensive response when criticized, easily offended

  o Eye contact that is intense, or no eye contact at all

  o Facial expressions, such as frowning or grimacing

  o Body language, such as clenching fists, waving arms

  o Rapid breathing

  o Aggressive postures, such as leaning forward, appearing tense

  o Verbal clues, such as loud, rapid talking

  o Drug or alcohol intoxication

Collaborative Care

- Nursing Care

  o Provide a safe environment not only for the client who is aggressive, but also for the other clients and staff on the unit.

  o Follow policies of the mental health setting when working with clients who demonstrate aggression.

○ Assess for triggers or preconditions that escalate client emotion.

○ Steps to handle aggressive and/or escalating behavior in a mental health setting include:

- Responding quickly

- Remaining calm and in control

- Encouraging the client to express feelings verbally, using therapeutic communication techniques (reflective techniques, silence, active listening)

- Allowing the client as much personal space as possible

- Maintaining eye contact and sitting or standing at the same level as the client

- Communicating with honesty, sincerity, and nonaggressive stance

- Avoiding accusatory or threatening statements

- Describing options clearly and offering the client choices

- Reassuring the client that staff are present to help prevent loss of control

- Setting limits for the client:

  □ Tell the client calmly and directly what he must do in a particular situation, such as, "I need you to stop yelling and walk with me to the day room where we can talk."

  □ Use physical activity, such as walking, to de-escalate anger and behaviors.

  □ Inform the client of the consequences of his behavior, such as loss of privileges.

- Use pharmacological interventions if the client does not respond to calm limit setting.

- Plan for four to six staff members to be available and in sight of the client as a "show of force" if appropriate.

○ Following an aggressive/violent episode:

- Discuss ways for the client to keep control during the aggression cycle.

- Encourage the client to talk about the incident and what triggered and escalated the aggression from the client's perspective.

- Debrief the staff to evaluate the effectiveness of actions.

- Document the entire incident completely by including:

  □ Behaviors leading up to, as well as those observed throughout the critical incident

  □ Nursing interventions implemented, and the client's response

- Medications
  - Haloperidol (Haldol)
    - Classification and therapeutic intent
      - Haloperidol is an antipsychotic agent used to control aggressive and impulsive behavior.
    - Nursing considerations
      - Monitor for signs and symptoms of parkinsonian and anticholinergic side effects.
  - Other medications may be used to prevent violent behavior by treating the underlying disorder. These include antidepressants, such as SSRIs; mood stabilizers, such as lithium; and sedative/hypnotic medications, such as benzodiazepines.
- Care After Discharge
  - Nursing Actions
    - Teach clients how to manage medications.
    - Assist the clients to develop problem-solving skills.
  - Client Education
    - Encourage clients to return for follow up.
    - Encourage clients to attend a support group.
- Client Outcomes
  - Client recognizes when feelings of anger occur and seeks appropriate assistance from staff.
  - Client takes responsibility for own actions.
  - Client is able to diffuse anger without losing control of behavior.
  - Client demonstrates appropriate problem-solving skills rather than violent behavior.

CHAPTER 29: ANGER MANAGEMENT

 Application Exercises

1. Which of the following statements made by a client is an example of aggressive communication?

    A. "I wish you would not make me angry."

    B. "I feel angry when you leave me."

    C. "It makes me angry when you interrupt me."

    D. "You'd better listen to me."

2. When approaching a client who is speaking in a loud voice with clenched fists, a nurse should

    A. insist that the client stop yelling.

    B. request other staff members to remain close by.

    C. move as close to the client as possible.

    D. walk away from the client.

3. A nurse is assessing a client in an inpatient mental health unit. Which of the following findings should the nurse expect if the client is in the preassaultive stage of violence?

    _____ Lethargy

    _____ Defensive responses to questions

    _____ Disorientation

    _____ Rapid breathing

    _____ Facial grimacing

    _____ Agitation

4. A client in the day room of an inpatient mental health setting gets up from a chair and throws it across the room. Which of the following is the priority nursing action?

    A. Encourage the client to express her feelings.

    B. Maintain eye contact with the client.

    C. Move the client away from others.

    D. Tell the client that the behavior is not acceptable.

CHAPTER 29: ANGER MANAGEMENT

 Application Exercises Answer Key

1. Which of the following statements made by a client is an example of aggressive communication?

A. "I wish you would not make me angry."

B. "I feel angry when you leave me."

C. "It makes me angry when you interrupt me."

D. "You'd better listen to me."

Using the words, "You'd better...," implies a threat (that something bad will happen if the person does not listen) and a lack of respect for the other individual. The other options do not imply a threat to, nor do they indicate a lack of respect of, another individual.

 NCLEX® Connection: Psychosocial Integrity: Therapeutic Communications

2. When approaching a client who is speaking in a loud voice with clenched fists, a nurse should

A. insist that the client stop yelling.

B. request other staff members to remain close by.

C. move as close to the client as possible.

D. walk away from the client.

In this situation, the nurse should request that other staff members remain close by to assist if necessary. The nurse should not make demands of the client by insisting that he stop yelling. This may further anger the client. Angry clients need a large personal space. The nurse should never walk away from an angry client. It is the nurse's responsibility to intervene as appropriate.

 NCLEX® Connection: Psychosocial Integrity: Behavioral Interventions

3. A nurse is assessing a client in an inpatient mental health unit. Which of the following findings should the nurse expect if the client is in the preassaultive stage of violence?

	Lethargy
X	**Defensive responses to questions**
	Disorientation
X	**Rapid breathing**
	Facial grimacing
X	**Agitation**

Defensive responses to questions, rapid breathing, and agitation are assessment findings that may indicate that a client is in the preassaultive stage of violence. Lethargy is more likely to be found in a client who is depressed. Disorientation is more likely to be found in a client who has a cognitive disorder.

 NCLEX® Connection: Psychosocial Integrity: Mental Health Concepts

4. A client in the day room of an inpatient mental health setting gets up from a chair and throws it across the room. Which of the following is the priority nursing action?

> A. Encourage the client to express her feelings.
>
> B. Maintain eye contact with the client.
>
> **C. Move the client away from others.**
>
> D. Tell the client that the behavior is not acceptable.

> **The greatest risk in this situation is harm to others. The priority action is for the nurse to move the client away from others to prevent injury.** Encouraging the client to express feelings, maintaining eye contact with the client, and telling the client that her behavior is not acceptable are all important interventions, but they are not the priority.

(N) NCLEX® Connection: Psychosocial Integrity: Behavioral Interventions

UNIT 6	PSYCHIATRIC EMERGENCIES
Chapter 30	Family and Community Violence

Overview

- Violence from one person toward another is a social act involving a serious abuse of power. Usually, a relatively stronger person controls or injures another, typically the least powerful person accessible to the abuser. This includes acts of violence committed by spouse against spouse, parent against child, or child against parent.

  o The nurse must be prepared to deal with various types of violence and the mental health consequences.

    ▪ Violence may be caused by a family member, a stranger, or an acquaintance, or it can come from a human-made mass-casualty incident, such as a terrorist attack.

    ▪ Natural disasters, such as hurricanes and earthquakes, can cause mental health effects comparable to those caused by human-made violence.

    ▪ Violence against a person with mental illness is more likely to occur when factors such as poverty, transient lifestyle, and substance abuse are present.

    ▪ A person with mental illness is no more likely to harm strangers than anyone else.

    ▪ The factor most likely to cause violence between strangers is a past history of violence and criminal activity.

Assessment

- Risk Factors

  o The female partner is the victim in the majority of family violence, but the male partner may also be a victim of violence.

  o Victims are at the greatest risk for violence when they try to leave the relationship.

  o Pregnancy tends to increase the likelihood of violence toward the domestic partner. The reason for this is unclear.

  o Factors that make abuse against children more likely include:

    ▪ The child is under 3 years of age.

    ▪ The child is perceived by the perpetrator as being different (the child is the result of an unwanted pregnancy, is physically disabled, or has some other trait that makes him particularly vulnerable).

(G)

- Older adults within the home may be abused because they are in poor health or because they exhibit disruptive behavior and because they are dependent on a caregiver. The potential for violence against an older adult is highest in families where violence has already occurred.

- Violence is most common within family groups, and most violence is aimed at family and friends rather than strangers.

  - Family violence occurs across all economic and educational backgrounds and racial/ethnic groups in the United States and is often termed "maltreatment."

  - Family violence/maltreatment can occur against children, domestic partners, or older adult family members.

  - Within the family, a cycle of violence can occur between domestic (intimate) partners:

    - Tension-building phase – The abuser has minor episodes of anger and may be verbally abusive and responsible for some minor physical violence. The victim is tense during this stage and tends to accept the blame for what is happening.

    - Serious battering phase – The tension becomes too much to bear and a serious incident takes place. The victim may try to cover up the injury or may get help.

    - Honeymoon phase – The situation is defused for awhile after the violent episode. The abuser becomes loving, promises to change, and is sorry for the behavior. The victim wants to believe this and hopes for a change. Eventually, the cycle begins again.

    - Periods of escalation and de-escalation usually continue with shorter and shorter periods of time between the two. Repeated episodes of violence lead to feelings of powerlessness.

- Cultural differences can influence whether or not the nursing assessment data is valid, how the client responds to interventions, and the appropriateness of nursing interactions with the client.

- Subjective and Objective Data

- Types of Violence

  - Physical violence occurs when pain or harm results:

    - Toward an infant or child, as is the case with shaken baby syndrome (caused by violent shaking of young infants)

    - Toward a domestic partner, such as striking or strangling the partner

    - Toward an older adult in the home (elder abuse), such as pushing an older adult parent and causing her to fall

  - Sexual violence occurs when sexual contact takes place without consent, whether the victim is able or unable to give that consent.

- ○ Emotional violence, which includes behavior that minimizes an individual's feelings of self-worth or humiliates, threatens, or intimidates a family member.

- ○ Neglect, which includes the failure to provide:

  - ■ Physical care, such as feeding

  - ■ The emotional care, such as interacting with a child, and/or stimulation necessary for a child to develop normally

  - ■ An education for a child, such as enrolling a young child in school

  - ■ Needed health or dental care

- ○ Economic maltreatment, which includes:

  - ■ Failure to provide the needs of a victim when adequate funds are available

  - ■ Unpaid bills, resulting in disconnection of heat or electricity

- ○ Victim characteristics

  - ■ Demonstration of low self-esteem and feelings of helplessness, hopelessness, powerlessness, guilt, and shame

  - ■ Attempts to protect the perpetrator and accept responsibility for the abuse

  - ■ Possible denial of the severity of the situation and feelings of anger and terror

- ○ Perpetrator characteristics

  - ■ Possible use of threats and intimidation to control the victim

  - ■ Is usually an extreme disciplinarian who believes in physical punishment

  - ■ Possible history of substance abuse

  - ■ Is likely to have experienced family violence as a child

- ○ Infants

  - ■ Shaken baby syndrome – Shaking may cause intracranial hemorrhage. Assess for respiratory distress, bulging fontanelles, and increased head circumference. Retinal hemorrhage may be present.

  - ■ Any bruising on an infant before age 6 months is suspicious.

  - ■ Preschoolers to adolescents

    - □ Assess for unusual bruising, such as on abdomen, back, or buttocks. Bruising is common on arms and legs in these age groups.

    - □ Assess the mechanism of injury, which may not be congruent with the physical appearance of the injury. Numerous bruises at different stages of healing may indicate continued beatings. Be suspicious of bruises or welts that have taken on the shape of a belt buckle or other object.

    - □ Assess for burns. Burns covering "glove" or "stocking" areas of the hands or feet may indicate forced immersion into boiling water. Small, round burns may be caused by lit cigarettes.

◻ Assess for fractures with unusual features, such as forearm spiral fractures, which could be caused by twisting the extremity forcefully. The presence of multiple fractures is suspicious.

◻ Assess for human bite marks.

◻ Assess for head injuries – level of consciousness, equal and reactive pupils, nausea/vomiting.

- Older adults

◻ Assess for any bruises, lacerations, abrasions, or fractures in which the physical appearance does not match the history or mechanism of injury.

Collaborative Care

- Nursing Care

  ○ All states have mandatory reporting laws that require nurses to report suspected abuse; there are civil and criminal penalties for not reporting suspicions of abuse.

  ○ Nursing interventions for child or older adult abuse must include the following:

    - Mandatory reporting of suspected or actual cases of child or older adult abuse

    - Complete, accurate documentation of subjective and objective data obtained during assessment

  ○ Conduct a nursing history.

    - Provide privacy when conducting interviews about family abuse.

    - Be direct, honest, and professional.

    - Use language the client understands.

    - Be understanding and attentive.

    - Use therapeutic techniques that demonstrate understanding.

    - Use open-ended questions to elicit descriptive responses.

    - Inform the client if a referral must be made to children's or adult protective services and explain the process.

  ○ Provide basic care to treat injuries.

  ○ Make appropriate referrals.

  ○ Nursing interventions for community-wide or mass casualty incidents include:

    - Early intervention

      ◻ Provide psychological first aid, which includes:

        ▸ Making sure the clients are physically and psychologically safe from harm

        ▸ Reducing stress-related symptoms, such as using techniques to alleviate a panic attack

        ▸ Providing interventions to restore rest/sleep and provide links to social supports and information about critical resources

- □ Depending on their level of expertise and training, mental health nurses may provide assessment, consultation, therapeutic communication and support, triage, and psychological/physical care.

- ■ Critical incident stress debriefing

    - □ This is a crisis intervention strategy used to assist individuals who have experienced a traumatic event, usually involving violence (staff experiencing client violence, school children and personnel experiencing the violent death of a student, rescue workers after an earthquake) in a safe environment.

    - □ Debriefing may take place in group meetings with a facilitator that and allows for a safe environment where thoughts and feelings may be expressed.

    - □ The facilitator will acknowledge reactions, provide anticipatory guidance for symptoms that may still occur, teach stress management techniques, and provide referrals.

    - □ The group may choose to meet on an ongoing basis or disband after resolution of the crisis.

- Care After Discharge

    - o Nursing Actions

        - ■ Help client develop a safety plan, identify behaviors and situations that might trigger violence and provide information regarding safe places to live.

        - ■ Encourage participation in support groups.

        - ■ Use case management to coordinate community, medical, criminal justice, and social services.

        - ■ Use crisis intervention techniques to help resolve family or community situations where violence has been devastating.

    - o Client Education

        - ■ Instruct clients regarding normal growth and development.

        - ■ Teach clients self-care and empowerment skills.

        - ■ Teach clients ways to manage stress.

- Client Outcomes

    - o Client will develop safety plan.

    - o Client will participate in self-help or support group.

    - o Client will identify strategies to manage stress.

    - o Client will be free from injury.

CHAPTER 30: FAMILY AND COMMUNITY VIOLENCE

 Application Exercises

Scenario: A nurse is visiting the home of a female client who has stage 5 Alzheimer's disease. The caregiver is the client's 35-year-old daughter, who also has three school-age children and a husband who travels most of each week. During the assessment, the nurse finds scattered bruising in the shape and size of handprints on the client's torso. When questioned, the caregiver states that the client was striking out at her and needed to be "quieted." The client is sleeping quietly, and the daughter states that she frequently needs to give her mother diazepam (Valium) to keep her calm.

1. What factors regarding the client and the home situation should alert the nurse to the possibility of abuse?

2. If the nurse is not sure that abuse has taken place, should she wait until another visit to gather more evidence before reporting her suspicions to adult protective services?

3. What is the nurse's responsibility in this situation and how should it be handled?

4. A nurse is assessing a preschool child in the emergency department. Which of the following findings should cause the nurse to suspect child abuse? (Select all that apply.)

_____ Scabs on knees

_____ Pinpoint burn marks on forearms

_____ Mismatched clothing

_____ Broken right arm

_____ Bruises on torso

CHAPTER 30: FAMILY AND COMMUNITY VIOLENCE

(A) Application Exercises Answer Key

Scenario: A nurse is visiting the home of a female client who has stage 5 Alzheimer's disease. The caregiver is the client's 35-year-old daughter, who also has three school-age children and a husband who travels most of each week. During the assessment, the nurse finds scattered bruising in the shape and size of handprints on the client's torso. When questioned, the caregiver states that the client was striking out at her and needed to be "quieted." The client is sleeping quietly, and the daughter states that she frequently needs to give her mother diazepam (Valium) to keep her calm.

1. What factors regarding the client and the home situation should alert the nurse to the possibility of abuse?

   Client factors: There are bruises in the shape of hand prints and the possibility that diazepam (Valium) may be used "to keep her calm" more often than necessary. The client has stage 5 Alzheimer's disease, which is moderate, or mid-stage, Alzheimer's disease, and is in the intermediate stage, which means she is quite confused and vulnerable.

   Caregiver factors: Caregiver role strain may be present, since the caregiver is also caring for three school-age children. She may lack support systems, since her husband is away during the week and she seems to be the only caregiver. More information is needed to assess both client and caregiver factors thoroughly.

   (N) NCLEX® Connection: Psychosocial Integrity: Abuse/Neglect

2. If the nurse is not sure that abuse has taken place, should she wait until another visit to gather more evidence before reporting her suspicions to adult protective services?

   No. As a professional, the nurse is liable and must report any suspicion of child or elder abuse.

   (N) NCLEX® Connection: Psychosocial Integrity: Abuse/Neglect

3. What is the nurse's responsibility in this situation and how should it be handled?

   The nurse has the responsibility to contact adult protective services if she suspects that any abuse has taken place. She must also make a decision about the client's safety regarding whether or not it is safe to keep the client in the home on the day of the visit. The nurse should thoroughly interview the caregiver, remaining calm, objective, understanding, and professional. Questions should be used that are open-ended and require a descriptive response so that they are less threatening and elicit more relevant information. The nurse should inform the daughter that a referral to adult protective services is necessary and explain the process. Documentation of the visit must be complete and accurate.

   (N) NCLEX® Connection: Psychosocial Integrity: Abuse/Neglect

4. A nurse is assessing a preschool child in the emergency department. Which of the following findings should cause the nurse to suspect child abuse? (Select all that apply.)

_____	Scabs on knees
X	**Pinpoint burn marks on forearms**
_____	Mismatched clothing
_____	Broken right arm
X	**Bruises on torso**

Pinpoint burn marks on the client's forearms may indicate burns caused by cigarettes, and bruises on the torso may indicate that the child has been beaten. Scabs on the client's knees, mismatched clothing, and a broken arm are expected findings that are consistent with the child's developmental age.

(N) NCLEX® Connection: Psychosocial Integrity: Abuse/Neglect

UNIT 6	PSYCHIATRIC EMERGENCIES
Chapter 31	Sexual Assault

Overview

- Sexual assault is defined as pressured or forced sexual contact, including sexually stimulated talk or actions, inappropriate touching or intercourse, incest, and rape (forced sexual intercourse).

- Rape is a crime of violence, aggression, anger, and power.

- The majority of rapists are known to the person who is raped.

- Reports of "date" or "acquaintance" rape have increased in recent years, often with drugs and alcohol used to facilitate the sexual assault. Drugs may include flunitrazepam (Rohypnol) and scopolamine (Burundanga).

- Most people who are raped suffer long-term and severe emotional trauma.

- Rape-trauma syndrome, which is similar to posttraumatic stress disorder, may occur after a rape.

Assessment

- Risk Factors

  - There is no "typical" rape survivor. Victims include individuals of all ages and can be either male or female.

- Subjective and Objective Data

  - Rape-trauma syndrome

    - Acute phase – Occurs immediately following the rape, lasts for about 2 weeks, and consists of the following:

      - Initial emotional reaction

        ‣ An expressed reaction is overt and consists of emotional outbursts, including crying, laughing, hysteria, anger, and incoherence.

        ‣ A controlled reaction is ambiguous; the survivor may appear calm and have blunted affect, but may also be confused, have difficulty making decisions, and feel numb.

      - A somatic reaction occurs later and lasts about 2 weeks. The client may have a variety of symptoms, including:

        ‣ Bruising and soreness from the attack

        ‣ Muscle tension, headaches, and sleep disturbances

- ▶ Gastrointestinal symptoms (nausea, anorexia, diarrhea, abdominal pain)

- ▶ Genitourinary symptoms (vaginal pain or discomfort)

- ▶ A variety of emotional reactions, including embarrassment, a desire for revenge, guilt, anger, fear, anxiety, and denial

- o Long-term reorganization phase occurs 2 weeks or more after the attack. Long-term psychological effects of sexual assault include:

  - Flashbacks and other intrusive thoughts about the assault

  - Increased activity, such as visiting friends frequently or moving residence, due to a fear that the assault will recur

  - Increased emotional responses (crying, anxiety, rapid mood swings)

  - Fears and phobias (fear of being alone, fear of sexual encounters)

  - Difficulties with daily functioning, low self-esteem, depression, sexual dysfunction, and somatic reports, such as headache or fatigue

- o Compound reaction

  - Reliance on alcohol or other drugs

  - Reactivated symptoms of previous conditions, such as physical or psychiatric illness

- o Silent reaction

  - Abrupt changes in relationships with partners

  - Nightmares

  - Increased anxiety during interview

  - Marked changes in sexual behavior

  - Sudden onset of phobic reactions

  - No verbalization of the occurrence of rape

- o Laboratory tests

  - Obtain blood for laboratory tests (HIV, hepatitis B and C).

  - Collect samples for legal evidence (hair, skin, semen).

Collaborative Care

- • Nursing Care

  - o Perform a self-assessment. It is vital that the nurse who works with the client who has been sexually assaulted be empathetic, objective, and nonjudgmental. If the nurse feels emotional about the assault due to some event or person in her own past, it may be better to allow another nurse to care for the client.

  - o Provide a private environment for an examination with a specially trained nurse-advocate, if available. A sexual assault nurse examiner (SANE) is a specially trained nurse who performs such examinations.

- ○ Provide nonjudgmental and empathetic care.

- ○ Obtain informed consent to collect data that can be used as legal evidence (photos, pelvic exam). The rape victim has the right to refuse either a medical examination or a legal exam, which provides forensic evidence for the police.

- ○ Treat any injuries and document care given.

- ○ Assist the specialist with the physical examination and the collection, documentation, and preservation of forensic evidence.

- ○ Support the client while legal evidence is being collected (samples of hair, skin, semen).

- ○ Administer prophylactic treatment for sexually transmitted diseases as outlined by the Centers for Disease Control and Prevention. This may include prophylactic treatment of syphilis, *Chlamydia*, and gonorrhea.

- ○ Evaluate for pregnancy risk and provide for prevention.

- ○ Call the client's available personal support system, such as a partner or parents, if the client gives permission.

- ○ Assist the client during the acute phase of rape-trauma syndrome to prepare for thoughts, symptoms, and emotions that may occur during the long-term phase of the syndrome.

  - ▪ Encourage the client to verbalize her story and her emotions.

  - ▪ Listen and let the survivor talk; use therapeutic techniques of reflection, open-ended questions, and active listening.

- • Care After Discharge

  - ○ Nursing Care

    - ▪ Provide phone numbers for 24-hr hotlines for rape survivors.

    - ▪ Promote of self-care activities: give follow-up instructions in writing, since the client may be unable to comprehend or remember verbal instructions.

    - ▪ Initiate referrals for needed resources and support services – Individual psychotherapy and group therapy may be helpful to increase coping skills and prevent long-term disability, such as depression, or suicidal ideation.

    - ▪ Schedule follow-up calls or visits at appropriate intervals after the assault.

- • Client Outcomes

  - ○ Client verbalizes feelings regarding assault.

  - ○ Client returns to regular daily activities.

  - ○ Client is free of somatic complaints.

  - ○ Client identifies support persons and ways to make contact.

CHAPTER 31: SEXUAL ASSAULT

 Application Exercises

1. A woman is brought to the emergency department by her roommate. The roommate says that she came home and found the client lying on the floor beaten and sexually assaulted. How should the nurse intervene with the client until the sexual assault nurse specialist arrives?

2. A rape victim states, "I never should have been out on the street alone at night." Which of the following is a therapeutic response by the nurse?

   A. "Your actions had nothing to do with what happened."

   B. "Blaming yourself only increases your anxiety and discomfort."

   C. "You believe this wouldn't have happened if you hadn't been out alone?"

   D. "You're right. You should not have been alone on the street at night."

3. A rape victim reports to the nurse that his family is not very supportive. Which of the following is a myth or belief about rape that might contribute to the family's response to the client?

   A. Rape is an act of aggression.

   B. No one asks to be raped.

   C. Men do not get raped.

   D. The majority of rapists are known to the victims.

4. A rape victim tells the emergency department nurse, "I feel so dirty. Please let me take a shower before anyone examines me. I just can't stand being so filthy!" How should the nurse respond?

   A. Arrange for the client to shower.

   B. Give the client a basin of hot water and towels.

   C. Explain that washing would destroy evidence.

   D. Ask the provider if the client can shower.

5. Rape-trauma syndrome is comparable to which of the following?

   A. Panic attack

   B. Disorganized schizophrenia

   C. Posttraumatic stress disorder

   D. Bipolar disorder

CHAPTER 31: SEXUAL ASSAULT

 Application Exercises Answer Key

1. A woman is brought to the emergency department by her roommate. The roommate says that she came home and found the client lying on the floor beaten and sexually assaulted. How should the nurse intervene with the client until the sexual assault nurse specialist arrives?

> Provide nonjudgmental care
> Assure the client that she is safe and that she did the right thing by coming to the emergency department.
> Provide privacy, but do not leave the client alone.
> Allow the roommate to stay, if the client wishes.
> Offer to call support persons.
> Do not allow the client to shower or otherwise clean up, so that evidence is preserved.
> Follow department/facility protocol.

 NCLEX® Connection: Psychosocial Integrity: Crisis Intervention

2. A rape victim states, "I never should have been out on the street alone at night." Which of the following is a therapeutic response by the nurse?

> A. "Your actions had nothing to do with what happened."
>
> B. "Blaming yourself only increases your anxiety and discomfort."
>
> **C. "You believe this wouldn't have happened if you hadn't been out alone?"**
>
> D. "You're right. You should not have been alone on the street at night."

By restating what the client said, the nurse is using the therapeutic technique of reflection to help the client verbalize her feelings. The other options give the nurse's opinion, and the nurse should remain nonjudgmental.

 NCLEX® Connection: Psychosocial Integrity: Therapeutic Communications

3. A rape victim reports to the nurse that his family is not very supportive. Which of the following is a myth or belief about rape that might contribute to the family's response to the client?

> A. Rape is an act of aggression.
>
> B. No one asks to be raped.
>
> **C. Men do not get raped.**
>
> D. The majority of rapists are known to the victims.

A fairly common myth is the notion that men do not experience sexual assault. The other options are true statements about sexual assault.

 NCLEX® Connection: Psychosocial Integrity: Mental Health Concepts

4. A rape victim tells the emergency department nurse, "I feel so dirty. Please let me take a shower before anyone examines me. I just can't stand being so filthy!" How should the nurse respond?

    A. Arrange for the client to shower.

    B. Give the client a basin of hot water and towels.

    C. Explain that washing would destroy evidence.

    D. Ask the provider if the client can shower.

Until evidence is collected and a physical examination is completed, the sexual assault survivor should not bathe or change clothes.

Ⓝ NCLEX® Connection: Psychosocial Integrity: Therapeutic Communications

5. Rape-trauma syndrome is comparable to which of the following?

    A. Panic attack

    B. Disorganized schizophrenia

    C. Posttraumatic stress disorder

    D. Bipolar disorder

Rape-trauma syndrome is comparable to posttraumatic stress disorder (PTSD), in which a person experiences or witnesses a threatening, horrific event. In PTSD, the person experiences stages of signs/symptoms including flashbacks, insomnia, anxiety, and many others. The other options are unlike rape-trauma syndrome in that they are either short-lived (panic attack) or are not precipitated by a traumatic event and do not occur in stages (schizophrenia and somatization disorder).

Ⓝ NCLEX® Connection: Psychosocial Integrity: Mental Health Concepts

References

Hockenberry, M. J., & Winkelstein M. L. (2009). *Wong's essentials of pediatric nursing* (8th ed.). St. Louis, MO: Mosby.

Lehne, R. A. (2010). *Pharmacology for nursing care* (7th ed.). St. Louis, MO: Saunders.

Roach, S. S., & Ford, S. M. (2008). *Introductory clinical pharmacology.* Philadelphia, PA: Lippincott Williams & Wilkins.

Townsend, M. C. (2008). *Essentials of psychiatric mental health nursing: Concepts of care in evidence-based practice* (4th ed.). Philadelphia, PA: F. A. Davis.

Varcarolis, E. M., Carson, V. B., & Shoemaker, N. C. (2006). *Foundations of psychiatric mental health nursing: A clinical approach* (5th ed.). St. Louis, MO: Saunders.

Wilson, B. A., Shannon, M. T., & Shields, K. M. (2010). *Pearson nurse's drug guide 2010.* Upper Saddle River, NJ: Prentice-Hall.